GW01237811

ALKALINE DIET COOKBOOK

250+ Recipes to Improve Your Health and Energy!

A Simple 30-Day Meal Plan for Beginners to Rebalance Your Metabolism, Including Anti-Inflammatory Recipes, Smoothies and Juices!

By

Lauren Smith

Table of Contents

Introduction

The alkaline diet is a plan with a partial or complete exclusion of foods that are "acidic". It's known that some foods form alkaline wastes after digestion and some turn into acidic toxins; acids tend to accumulate in the body, which can lead to acid-base balance disorder, the development of various diseases, and the acceleration of the aging processes. The human body has a physiological tendency to oxidize; for normal functioning, **the body needs to maintain an acid-base balance of blood and tissues**. Even minor deviation from the acid-base balance norm (7.35 - 7.45) can be life-threatening. However, it's totally possible to control tissues oxidation with the help of food. **It's enough to add more alkalizing foods into your daily menus and reduce foods that increase acidity**. The alkaline diet isn't new: the benefits of this diet were proven by Otto Barburg back in 1932. This scientist discovered that cancer cells were particularly active in acidic environments. Acid-base balance is also supported by modern scientists: the normal balance of our blood is "shifted" to the alkaline side, with a pH level slightly higher than 7. Doctors formerly recommended this diet to patients who suffered from joint pain, gout, and high acidity of their digestion systems. It's believed that this particular diet yields the best results, as it helps to lose and maintain weight. It's one of the safest diets for health.

Acidic Versus Neutral Products

The pH imbalance in the body can be caused by acidic foods that usually dominate in the daily menu. To minimize the risk of a Ph imbalance, you need to limit the consumption of meat, poultry, fish (trout and salmon are allowed), seafood, cottage cheese, milk, animal fat, lard, fast foods, eggs, white rice, wheat, beans, dried peas, mushrooms, cashew nuts, sesame seeds, and peanuts. Sunflower seeds are also considered as an acidic product.

Ketchup and mustard can also cause a Ph imbalance. In addition, you must exclude all pastries made from white flour from your menu, as well as sweets, including honey. Coffee, soda drinks, and most alcoholic beverages also lead to increased acidity. **According to nutritionists, 80 percent of the food you consume must be alkaline, and only 20 can be acid!**

However, in our daily diet, it's also important to consider one more factor: foods aren't only divided into acid and alkaline, but there's actually a third category. It includes foods with an acid and alkali combination. This list contains vegetable oil, rye bread, whole grain products, and cereals.

Some foods, also, can affect the body in different ways: in one case they can form acid, and in some cases, they can form alkali. Thus, you should be careful with the consumption of sour milk, melon, apricots, currants, gooseberries, and kiwi.

The experts who first suggested an alkaline diet for healthier living say that acidic metabolic waste is harmful to bodily health as it can disrupt the optimal pH levels within the body, which are essential to regulating enzyme function, hormone production, and other metabolic reactions. That is why the alkaline diet was proposed; it can help maintain the internal alkaline environment by producing alkaline metabolic waste.

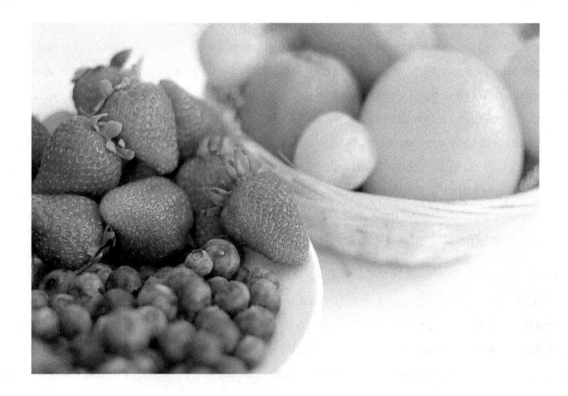

What Is The Alkaline Diet?

The Alkaline Diet, or the Alkaline Ash Diet, takes a whole new approach to what we consume. It does not consider the proportions or the nutritional composition of foods like other diets do. Instead, it considers the effects the different types of metabolic waste produce after food has been digested and assimilated. **The type of food determines the nature of its metabolic waste**. Therefore, food containing acid compounds or acidic elements produces acidic waste, whereas alkaline foods produce alkaline metabolic waste. Acidic metabolic waste is harmful to bodily health because it can disrupt the body's optimal pH levels, which are essential to regulating enzyme function, hormone production, and other metabolic reactions. The scientists discovered that following an alkaline diet, your body produces alkaline metabolic waste and can maintain a healthier environment.

What is pH?

Put simply, a pH value defines the measure of alkalinity, or basicity and acidity, of a substance or an environment. There is an optimal pH value required to carry out basic metabolic functions. On the scale of 0-14, substances with 0-6 pH values are considered acidic, those having 7 are neutral, and ones with 8-14 pH values are basic in nature. Human blood is also slightly alkaline, having a value of 7.35-7.45 on the pH scale. This pH value is optimal for all the components carried by the blood in the body. Since blood is pivotal to all metabolic functions in the body, it carries hormones, enzymes, nutrients, and other essential substances, it important to maintain the necessary pH level.

How Does Food Affect Your Body?

As we have discussed, optimal pH is vital to support normal metabolic functions. When we eat substances that can produce acidic by-products or end products, they will likely end up in our blood and may lower its pH value, making it more acidic. Once that balance is disrupted, all the functions associated with the blood and the components present in it are also slowed down, or they are not properly executed in the body. Moreover, acidic foods can also be harmful to the microbes residing in the human intestine as they require a high pH level to survive. Contrarily, if we eat foods that can support a normal pH level in the body, whether in the blood or in the cells, it can be very healthy for us.

How Does the Alkaline Diet Help?

The principle on which the alkaline diet works is simple: do not eat foods which are considered acid-forming or acidic. It means that substances which have a tendency to produce acidic metabolic waste or by-products should be avoided to maintain natural pH levels in the body. Even when it comes to digestion, it is only the stomach that digests food in an acidic environment; the same food has to be transformed into an alkaline state before reaching the intestines for complete digestion and assimilation. The alkaline diet, therefore, recommends consuming foods which produce alkaline metabolic waste or end products.

Proof That the Alkaline Diet is Useful

A 2010 cancer study suggests that acidic food can hinder the successful treatment of cancer while depriving the body of its optimal metabolic conditions (Diet and cancer prevention: Contributions from the European Prospective Investigation into Cancer and Nutrition (EPIC) study- Carlos A. Gonzalez, 2010). Experts discovered that when cancer patients were given alternative alkaline diets, they became healthier and more resilient against the disease. Similarly, there is evidence from a 2017 study that tells us about the harm an acidic diet can have and how it can negatively affect kidney health- (Reducing the Dietary Acid Load: How a More Alkaline Diet Benefits Patients with Chronic Kidney Disease- Carolina Passey, 2017). In contrast to this, the alkaline diet has not only proven effective in preventing kidney problems, but it is also good for heart health, regulation of hormones, and boosting brain function.

The Microbiome and its Role in Alkalinity

The microbiome is a whole community of microbes that live inside the human digestive system. We are familiar with the fact that there are numerous nutrients which cannot be digested by human-produced enzymes. These microbes present in the gut help us digest those nutrients and break them down into simpler components. These microbes can survive only in an alkaline environment and, therefore, they also produce alkaline by-products to maintain the pH around them: that is why they are both contributors to and beneficiaries from this alkalinity. Also, when we eat acid-forming food, it is likely to disturb this naturally occurring microbiome.

The Ratio of Macros and How that Affects Alkalinity

Every macronutrient has a different composition; some carry more acidic components than others. Proteins, for example, have amino acids as their monomers (the basic molecular structure which makes up a protein chain) that are acidic in nature. Overconsumption of complex proteins, like those present in red meat, can likely affect the body's alkalinity level. On the other hand, less complex amino acids are not completely restricted in the alkaline diet, in which it is important the quality of protein intake. Although carbohydrates usually contain fewer acids, foods containing carbohydrates are considered acid-forming. Fats have fatty acids that can also negatively affect alkalinity, especially animal fats, which are restricted on the alkaline diet.

How to Follow the Alkaline Diet

Follow the alkaline diet is simple: eat more alkaline foods. Alkaline Diet could improve health conditions. Some of the conditions and problems in which the alkaline diet can complement medical treatment and therapies could be:

- Diabetes
- Muscle Pain
- Gout
- Arthritis
- Bloating
- Cancer
- Insomnia

What is Alkaline Water?

Pure water is neutral, and it has a pH value of 7. Alkaline water, on the other hand, has a higher value of 8 to 9 on the pH scale. This water can be consumed to help maintain alkalinity within the human body, especially the gut and blood. It is used for various purposes, from detoxification to countering the effects of aging, reducing obesity, and fighting cancer.

Alkaline Diet Frequently Asked Questions

Q. What is the difference between alkaline food and the Acid Reflux diet?

The acid reflux diet is mainly concerned with the role of the stomach and its proper functioning. This diet was created to reduce the acidity in the stomach and stop the overproduction of hydrochloric acid (HCl) in the stomach. However, the alkaline diet is focused on the pH balance within the body, whether it is in the gut, blood, or other organs.

Q. How can alkaline food control obesity?

The alkaline diet recommends a reduction in intake of complex carbs, sugars, and saturated fats. All these food items are mainly responsible for obesity.

Q. Does cooking change the alkalinity of food?

No, this is far from reality. The acidic and basic character of the food is its chemical property, it does not change during overheating or cooking.

Alkaline and Acid-Forming Foods

The food we eat can be categorized into two main groups with respect to the alkaline diet. The one which has the tendency to produce acidic metabolic waste and is known as acid-forming, whereas the food which can produce alkaline metabolic products after digestion is known as an alkaline-forming food. Let's take a look and categorize different ingredients on the basis of this property.

Acid-Forming Foods

- Coffee and other caffeinated drinks
- Beef, pork, lamb, fish, and chicken
- Popcorn
- Cornmeal, rye
- Rice: white, brown, or basmati
- Wheat germ
- Colas
- Cheese
- Pasta
- Alcoholic drinks
- Soy sauce
- Ketchup
- Sweetened yogurt
- Mustard
- Refined table salt
- Mayonnaise
- Tobacco
- White vinegar
- Nutmeg

Alkalinizing Foods

- Peas
- Beans: string, soy, lima, green, and snap
- Arrowroot flour
- Grains: flax, millet, quinoa, and amaranth
- Potatoes
- Nuts: almonds, pignolia, fresh coconut, and chestnuts
- Sprouted seeds of alfalfa, radish, and chia
- Unsprouted sesame
- Fresh unsalted butter
- Whey
- Plain yogurt
- Fruit juices
- All vegetable juices

- Most herbal teas
- Garlic
- Cayenne pepper
- Gelatin
- Most herbs
- Miso
- Most vegetables
- Unprocessed sea salt
- Most spices
- Vanilla extract
- Sweeteners: raw, unpasteurized honey, dried sugar cane juice (Sucanat), brown rice syrup
- Brewer's yeast

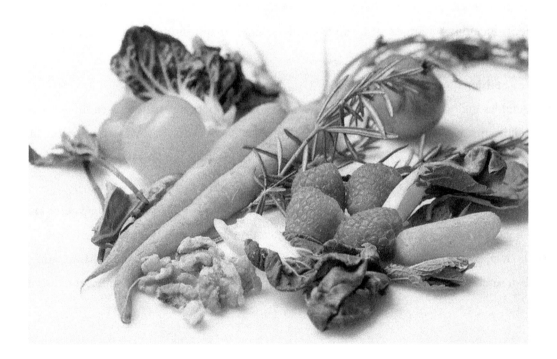

Foods to Eat

For the most part, fruits and vegetables are considered alkaline, while meat, dairy, and highly processed foods are viewed to be more acid-forming. The concern is that high levels of acid ash in the body overtax the body's acid-base regulatory mechanisms, which disrupts other regulatory functions in the body. Luckily, your body is more capable of regulating blood pH than you think. We have not yet entirely understood the etiology in which highly inflammatory conditions, such as kidney disease, but scientific researches discovered that Alkaline Foods are good for health primarily because they are plant foods. Indeed, plant foods contain a wide variety of essential vitamins, minerals, amino acids, and antioxidants: they provide a synergy of nutritional benefits, in their whole form. Let's take a look at some.

Dark Leafy Greens

Dark leafy greens include kale, spinach, chard, arugula, and green-leaf and romaine lettuce. They deliver an array of nutrients including vitamins A, C, and K, folate, fiber, magnesium, calcium, iron, and potassium.

Non-Starchy Vegetables

Non-starchy vegetables include radishes, mushrooms, artichokes, asparagus, broccoli, cauliflower, cucumber, carrots, jicama, peppers, and, of course, leafy greens. They come in a variety of colors and textures, and like leafy greens, they provide very few calories per gram of weight.

Fruits

When we consider fruits, we are looking at plant foods that not only provide a naturally sweeter taste, but also contain a variety of antioxidant nutrients and essential vitamins and minerals. Fruits are delicious on their own, paired with nuts or nut butters, in salads and healthy green smoothies, and even added as natural sweeteners to balance out flavors in bitter greens like arugula and some savory dishes like curries.

Nuts

Although nuts are high in calories, they offer healthy monounsaturated and polyunsaturated fatty acids such as omega-3s that are essential for brain function and hormonal regulation in the body. So, include these in your diet, but exercise portion control—1 ounce (2 tablespoons) is considered one serving. Nuts provide nutrients such as magnesium (which helps regulate blood pressure) and immune-supportive vitamin E. According to research, nuts may help lower bad cholesterol, lower levels of inflammation related to heart disease, and improve the structure and lining of your arteries. The

American Heart Association suggests consuming 1.5 ounces (3 tablespoons) of unsalted nuts per day, four times per week.

Seeds

Like nuts, seeds are also calorie-dense but full of nutrients. They also provide polyunsaturated and monounsaturated fats, as well as fiber and nutrients like vitamin E. Consumed in small portions, they can be part of a healthy diet. Like nuts, seeds may help regulate blood sugar (as they are low in carbohydrates and include dietary fiber) and blood pressure. Top your salads or soups with a light sprinkling of seeds to provide a delicate crunch, a bit of flavor, and some added nutrients to your plate.

Olive Oil and Avocado Oil

These oils are included in your healthy fats because they can help provide you with the essential fatty acids you need. The monounsaturated and polyunsaturated fats in these healthy oils benefit the brain, nerves, skin, nails, and hormonal regulation, too! Used sparingly to lightly coat leafy greens (and when used in combination with spices and other foods), they help carry and distribute flavor to your palate.

Beans and Other Legumes

These plant foods are special because they are not only rich in complex carbohydrates, but also good sources of protein, making them a part of two food groups. Additionally, they are rich sources of fiber and essential B vitamins.

Whole Grains

Intact whole grains such as quinoa and buckwheat provide some protein, as well as the benefit of complex carbohydrates, and their fiber content ultimately assists in blood sugar control. They bring B vitamins to the table, as well as a variety of other heart-healthy nutrients, including iron, magnesium, and phosphorus.

Tofu and Soybeans

Soybeans (known as edamame in their whole, cooked form) can be processed into tofu, which, like its base component, is a good protein source. Yes, tofu is processed, but not highly processed, and thus it doesn't contain a lot of additives. Generally, it is made up of three ingredients: soybeans, water, and a coagulant. Tofu offers the benefit of a convenient source of protein that can easily translate into many different dishes due to the variety of textures available and its mild flavor.

Apple Cider Vinegar

This vinegar is highly touted in many popularized versions of the alkaline diet. The benefit of this tangy acid (which, like lemon, leaves an alkaline ash in the body) is that its flavor is so intense, just a little can add a lot of flavor to your food. As a fermented food, it may help support digestive health.

Foods to Avoid

Although this diet is not highly restrictive, there is a very good reason to limit or avoid certain foods. Many of the following foods are not only more acidic, they are also more inflammatory, especially if consumed in large amounts. Even though some of the foods on this list provide some nutritional benefit (e.g., meat is a protein-rich food that contains the essential vitamin B12), it is best to focus more on your fruits, veggies, intact whole grains, beans, and legumes. Below are some reasons, beyond their acidity, to limit or avoid the following foods.

Red Meat

Red meat contains phosphorus, an essential nutrient you can also obtain from plant foods. It is also a very good source of protein and vitamin B12. However, it is higher in saturated fat than other proteins, such as chicken, fish, and vegetable proteins. Saturated fats have been correlated with cardiovascular disease risk factors. There is strong evidence that consuming red meat and processed meats causes cancer, particularly colorectal cancer, according to the American Institute for Cancer Research, and a large body of scientific evidence links the high intake of red meat and processed meats to greater risks of heart disease, cancer, and diabetes, according to Harvard Health.

Processed Meats

Processed meats include sausages, ham, corned beef, smoked meats, and dried meats, which are preserved through curing, salting, smoking, or drying. High intake of processed meats has been implicated in chronic disease, including high blood pressure, cancer, and heart disease.

Added Sugars

Added sugars include, but are not limited to, refined white sugar, brown sugar, corn syrup, rice syrup, dextrose, honey, malt sugar, and molasses—many of which are found in highly processed foods. Diets high in added sugars are widely known to promote insulin resistance and weight gain. Scientific evidence also reveals that high sugar intake can increase cardiovascular risk, including raising triglycerides and LDL ("bad") cholesterol and promoting inflammation, blood platelet disruption, and oxidative stress that contributes to atherosclerosis (hardening of the arteries).

Dairy

Dairy includes milk, yogurt, kefir, butter, and any of those foods processed from the milk of an animal (e.g., cow and goat milk). Many dairy foods have the benefit of containing calcium and protein, and some, such as yogurt and kefir, contain probiotics. Dairy can contribute to allergies or sensitivities in certain individuals, and some science supports that it can be inflammatory in the body (although there is conflicting evidence on this matter). Regardless, limiting dairy is not detrimental, as you can get plenty of calcium and protein from a wide variety of plant foods.

Highly Processed Grains

Highly processed grains include breads, muffins, crackers, tortillas, cakes, and pastries. The processing of wheat, rice, and other whole grains into flour (an ingredient in these foods) removes the outer fiber-rich layer and nutrient-dense germ, leaving behind the starch, which is rapidly converted to sugar in the body—a process that can adversely affect blood sugar. Furthermore, highly processed foods contain additives, including sugars, sodium, chemicals, stabilizers, and more, that have little benefit for the body, and some of these (like BHT added as a preservative) are considered toxic. Additionally, some unexpired, highly processed foods may contain trans fats if they were manufactured before 2018, when the fats were banned.

Alcohol

Wine, beer, vodka, and gin are broad examples of alcohol people may enjoy. Studies implicate excessive alcohol intake with blood pressure and heart disease risk. Furthermore, many alcoholic drinks include added sugars or syrups—further increasing the sugar content of the drink.

Coffee

Caffeine may be beneficial for its immediate energy boost, but these effects don't last long. Studies that support its health contributions (as well as deficits to optimal health) are conflicting. Dependency on caffeine can reduce intake of nutrient-dense options if you use it constantly to boost your energy to get through the day.

Chocolate

When we refer to chocolate, we are generally not talking about the cocoa bean itself, but rather the product it gets processed into, whether it's chocolate chips, a chocolate bar, or cocoa powder for hot cocoa. Consuming sugar-free chocolate is not much better; many people feel that artificial sweeteners give you permission to consume more artificially flavored foods with less nutritional value. Not only does the chocolate we eat contain added sugars or sugar substitutes, it's also calorie-dense and contains caffeine.

Soda

Sodas are often processed with added sugars or sugar substitutes (non-nutritive sweeteners). Sugar substitutes are highly processed and may not have the overall health benefits one might expect, despite containing little to no calories or sugars. Furthermore, sodas don't provide much nutritional value beyond the phosphorus they contain (which actually may be excessive for anyone who overconsumes soda). Additionally, soda is a diuretic and thus dehydrating. Drinking soda to quench thirst is actually counterproductive, as it often replaces necessary recommended water intake.

Protein Supplements

Protein supplements include blends of vegetable proteins such as pea protein or animal-derived proteins such as whey protein or collagen. It is important to note that many of these powders or blends are highly processed. Although some supplements may contain a convenient source of protein (and perhaps other additional nutrients), they are highly processed and thus exposed to chemicals used in the processing. It is better to get your nutrients from whole foods.

The 80/20 Approach

This alkaline diet book is not limited only to highly alkaline foods; rather, it follows an 80/20 rule. This means you can enjoy a wide variety of foods in the alkaline spectrum, while allowing for foods that fall in the acidic range. **Enjoying 80 percent alkaline foods and 20 percent acidic foods makes this diet realistic and unrestrictive**. I think an overly restrictive diet can set people up for failure. Did you know that two out of five people quit a diet after just seven days? Eighty percent fail to remain on a diet for more than a month. Lifestyle changes are more likely to stick when we don't feel any deprivation. Depending on your overall health goal, cheats can include a 5-ounce glass of red wine, a 2½-inch chocolate chip cookie, or even a 3-ounce piece of steak. Furthermore, some very healthy, nutritious foods such as barley, buckwheat, bulgur wheat, kidney beans, pinto beans, and even heart-healthy omega-3-rich walnuts fall within the acidic range. These foods help you meet your protein needs and fiber requirements and provide specific nutrients that you might otherwise miss in a restrictive alkaline diet. We wouldn't want you to lose out on the nutritional benefits of these foods.

5 Myths About the Alkaline Diet

There are many myths about the alkaline diet. Here are the most common, and the truth behind them.

You Have to Drink Alkaline Water

You don't have to drink only alkaline water. Much of the science that supports this assertion is funded by companies that market this product. As with food, there is no substantial scientific evidence to support that alkaline water or drinks will change your blood pH. According to a 2016 systematic review published in BMJ, despite the promotion of the alkaline diet and alkaline water to support cancer treatment, there is a lack of scientific evidence to substantiate this claim. More than 8,000 citations were identified and over 250 abstracts reviewed for this scientific analysis.

You Have to Take Supplements

While following the alkaline diet, some people have concerns about getting enough B12, calcium, iron, vitamin D, and protein. Fortunately, you can get enough of all these from the following healthy, natural sources:
- *B12*: nutritional yeast, fortified soymilk, tofu
- *Calcium*: almonds, broccoli, strawberries, beans, peas, lentils, soybeans, chia seeds, flaxseed
- *Iron*: lentils, chickpeas, tofu, cashews, chia seeds, apricots, kale, raisins, quinoa (combining these iron-rich foods with a source of vitamin C such as oranges or strawberries will improve iron absorption in the body)

- *Vitamin D*: sunlight is a free source of vitamin D (according to research, you only need 10 minutes of sun exposure per day to promote the production of vitamin D in the body); you can also obtain it from mushrooms and fortified plant-based milks
- *Protein:* soymilk, soybeans, beans and legumes, nuts, seeds, and a wide variety of leafy greens and non-starchy vegetables for their varying amino acid compositions

Some supplements can be helpful, but it really depends on individual needs. For example, B12 deficiencies are easily masked by high intake of folate (highly present in plant foods). Nutritional yeast fortified with B12 is considered a good source for vegans, as 1 tablespoon can provide as much as 5 micrograms of B12 (that's approximately twice the RDA for adult men and non-pregnant, non-lactating women). And although sunlight is a free source of vitamin D, some individuals have more susceptibility for inadequate absorption. Additionally, multivitamin supplementation is beneficial to any individual, especially adults over 50 who are at increased risk of poorer absorption of nutrients from food. Although supplementation isn't a must for everyone who follows a healthy alkaline diet, it can be beneficial.

You Can't Eat Any Meat or Fish

There are many variations of the alkaline diet, some stricter than others. Most alkaline diets have an 80/20 or 70/30 rule, allowing for some flexibility to include a small percentage of meat or fish. Specific nutrients may be difficult to obtain from a strictly vegan diet. These include B12 (which is more actively available in animal sources) and certain forms of omega-3s that are not present in plant foods. Fatty fish, such as salmon, is recommended, as it is a direct source of eicosapentaenoic acid (EPA), an essential Omega-3. Therefore, I'm providing you with some things to consider regarding whether you choose to include these in your healthy alkaline diet.

It's Dangerous

No particular food or drink can change your blood pH, so you are not at risk for alkalosis by following an alkaline diet. According to the Merck Manual, metabolic alkalosis is a manifestation of extreme fluid and electrolyte losses (i.e., sodium and potassium) that can occur as a result of excessive vomiting, kidney malfunction, overactive adrenals, or diuretics. However, those who place strict emphasis on solely alkaline foods can be at risk for nutrient deficiencies. (This healthy alkaline diet does not promote such exclusivity.) Furthermore, excessive food restriction can lead to unhealthy relationships with food (eating disorders), as well as some symptoms that may occur in anorexic individuals, including amenorrhea (lack of menstrual periods) and risk factors for heart arrhythmia (alarmingly low heart rate and blood pressure). When it comes to potential nutrient deficiencies, through a well-planned alkaline diet (which is essentially vegan), you can obtain all your essential nutrients. However, depending on the individual, supplementation may be necessary.

The Alkaline Diet Is Just a Weight-Loss Diet

Weight loss may be a desired side effect of the alkaline diet. However, the intent and overall design of this whole food, plant-based diet is to deliver optimal health conditions for disease risk prevention. Limiting red meats, dairy, and highly processed foods in favor of higher intakes of fruits and vegetables usually leads to weight loss because plant foods are lower in calories but high in nutrient density and dietary fiber—all factors that promote blood sugar control, satiety, and, ultimately, weight loss.

Benefits of The Alkaline Diet

No matter what type of food is someone's favorite food, there is a diet plan that revolves around it; so many diets are going around today that it is difficult to know which one is the best! But the best diet for eliminating and avoiding disease and promoting a long and healthy life is the alkaline diet. Researchers have discovered that just by balancing the body's pH level through a diet of the proper foods for optimum health, a host of ailments can be eliminated or avoided before they begin. The way the alkaline diets works is quite simple. A diet that features predominantly highly alkaline foods allows the body to maintain a more alkaline pH level; this allows the body to use its own natural processes to protect the healthy cells and maintain a good balance of essential minerals to proper body functioning. This is especially important for people who use fasting as a way to lose or maintain weight, because fasting can alter hormone levels in the body, and the alkaline diet will help maintain proper hormone levels.

Adding on excessive weight is one of the ways that the body tries to adapt to a high level of acidity. Humans produce acids constantly just by being alive. If the diet people consume is loaded with acid producing drinks and foods, then the body's natural ability to adapt to dietary changes is overloaded and damaged. If the acids are not being excreted through the body's waste, then the body will begin to store the acids in the fatty tissue. One of the kidneys' main functions is to excrete waste products in the urine it creates. Excess body acid is one of these waste products. Some of the hormones in the body, like Cortisol, will work to help the kidneys excrete excess acid. Cortisol is one of the major factors that lead to excess fat stores in the body called visceral fat, which is stored around the body's internal organs. It also leads to excessive stores of fat in the abdomen. The problem with the body's cortisol production is that it doesn't always happen when it is most needed. The adrenal glands will produce extra amounts of the hormones cortisol and adrenaline whenever the brain perceives that the body is under stress, such as when someone is physically attacked. The problem is that the brain cannot distinguish between real stress that is immediate in nature and stress caused by other problems in the body. Of course, a physical attack would cause feelings of stress, but there are things humans do to themselves that will cause the body to feel stressed enough to release excess amounts of cortisol. Some of these might include:

- Overwork
- Being overweight
- Struggling to walk with joints hampered by excess weight
- Inability to breathe well because of excess weight
- High blood pressure
- Underlying diseases like diabetes or kidney disease

The list could go on and on. The point is that anything that causes the body to feel stress will cause the body to release excess amounts of cortisol above what is needed for optimum cell function.

Cortisol has specific functions in the body: it is a necessary chemical in the workings of the human body. It helps to regulate energy by selecting either protein, fat, or carbohydrate to fuel the body's need, and it is also responsible for providing the cells with glucose for energy when the need arises. Cortisol also works to inhibit the production of insulin by the pancreas. Every cell in the body has a cortisol receptor. Problems start when there is an excess of cortisol in the body as there is in times of stress. Remember that the body is unable to tell the difference between real stress from an outside source and manufactured stress from poor health habits. So, for example, when the body continuously makes more cortisol, the pancreas makes more insulin to act against the cortisol. Eventually the cells of the body stop responding to the insulin and only respond to the cortisol, which makes the body store excess fat in places it should not store excess fat. The pancreas stops producing insulin, the sugar levels in the blood stream rise and stay high, and the person develops Type 2 Diabetes along with being overweight. Both of these conditions cause the body to put out an ever-increasing amount of acid that the body then needs to struggle to get rid of.

The alkaline diet can reverse this vicious cycle or prevent it from ever happening in the first place by helping to maintain a proper weight. By focusing on the consumption of healthy foods and the elimination of foods that cause excess amounts of acid production in the body, the alkaline diet helps restore the balance of cortisol and insulin in the body, reducing weight and reversing the effects of diabetes on the body. By following the alkaline diet and eating alkaline foods it is natural to stop consuming foods that add high amounts of acid to the body. This will begin to give the body the break it needs from excess amount of acid. Since a chronic elevation of cortisol results in a chronic elevation of sugar levels in the blood, this can lead to health problems throughout the body. Some of these health issues include a loss of cognitive functioning, increased fat accumulation, loss of muscle mass, high blood pressure, depressed immune functions, and a loss of calcium from bones.

When the alkaline diet is followed regularly, the cortisol levels in the bloodstream will begin to return to normal, and the pancreas can begin to produce insulin in the correct amounts again. Once this happens, the body will prompt the liver to release a chemical stored there called glycogen, which is nothing more than blood sugar stored in the liver to be used for energy and fuel for the cells in the body. Once there is no longer excess sugar in the body, the body will turn to the liver to release its stored glycogen. Once the stores in the liver have been depleted, the body will turn to stored fat to burn as fuel and energy for the cells of the body and the systems of the body. And when this happens weight loss will occur.

Getting and keeping the level of blood sugar back to normal and losing weight will improve quality of life. But the alkaline diet has other health benefits for the body besides weight loss.

Weight loss is essential because excess weight and cardiovascular disease work hand in hand in the body. Besides being at risk for other cardiovascular diseases, obese people have a higher risk of developing heart failure. This happens because of several factors. Excess body fat causes the body to have a higher volume of blood, since the body needs more blood to circulate through the body and take nutrients to all of the cells. This higher volume of blood causes the heart to work harder, since it has more blood to pump through to process. Excessive deposits of fat stored in the body, especially those stored in the stomach area, release many harmful toxins and inflammatory chemicals that cause damage to the muscles of the heart, and it is not necessary to have symptoms of heart disease actually to have heart disease. Excess body weight is also responsible for casing high blood pressure; this goes along with the increased volume of blood in the body. The extra fat tissue needs nutrients and oxygen in order to survive, and the systems of the body are not in the habit of starving one of their own. More blood circulating through the body causes extra pressure on the walls of the arteries and veins that the blood must pass through. This higher pressure is what causes high blood pressure: as the blood continues to funnel through the fat deposits, it will pick up fat molecules and drop them off at other places in the body. These fat deposits latch onto the arteries' walls and form thick places that make it nearly impossible for the blood to flow freely, a condition is known as atherosclerosis or hardening of the arteries. This hardening leads to coronary artery disease. When these fat deposits break loose and flow through the bloodstream, they can cause a heart attack. Moreover, being obese places an enormous amount of pressure on the joints of the hips and the knees. One pound of excess weight places four pounds of extra pressure on the joints in the lower half of the body, pressure these joints were not built to withstand for a long period. Over time these joints can become so damaged by obesity that the only cure is a complete joint replacement. However, joint replacement is usually not done on obese people because of the risk of complications and the poor rate of successful recovery.

The alkaline diet can significantly reduce the amount of strain placed on the body's natural detoxification systems. Eating alkaline food will create an environment that is more ideal for body's cells to grow in while it works to support it with good nutrition and strengthen the body's natural immunity. Moreover, the alkaline diet can be beneficial to the kidneys also, that they work hard to help regulate the pH level of the blood in the body by removing toxins from the body's cells. People with kidney disease will have a harder time removing waste products through the kidneys. The alkaline diet could assist in rebalancing the body's pH level and thus easing some of the kidney's burdens. The acid we eat from acid food is stored in the body and leads to a weakening of the body's muscles and bones.

Breakfast Recipes

1. Good Morning Popeye

Preparation Time: 5 minutes

Cooking Time: 10 minutes

Servings: 2

Ingredients:

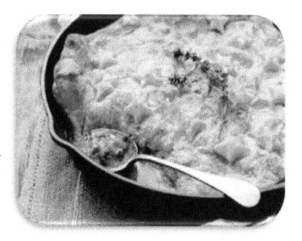

- 1 Tbsp coconut oil
- 2 medium sweet potatoes, peeled and cubed
- 1 medium sweet onion, chopped
- 1 red bell pepper, seeded, chopped
- ¼ cup sliced mushrooms, any type
- 2 garlic cloves, chopped
- 4 cups spinach
- 1 tsp onion powder
- 1 tsp garlic powder
- ½ tsp Bouquet Garni herb blend, or other dried herbs such as rosemary or sage
- ½ tsp sea salt

Directions:

1. In a medium bowl, combine the oil, sweet potatoes, onion, red bell pepper, mushrooms, garlic, spinach, onion powder, garlic powder, Bouquet Garni, and salt.
2. Toss the vegetables in the oil until evenly coated.
3. Heat a nonstick frying pan over medium heat and cook the vegetables, stirring, for 10 minutes, or until tender.
4. Divide into two portions and serve.

Nutrition:

Carbohydrates – 37.8 g

Fiber – 8.1 g

Fat – 1.5 g

Protein – 5.6 g

Calories – 181

2. Garden Pancakes

Preparation Time: 5 minutes

Cooking Time: 5 minutes

Servings: 2

Ingredients:

- 1 medium zucchini, roughly chopped
- 1 carrot, peeled and roughly chopped
- 1 yellow squash, roughly chopped
- ½ small white onion, grated
- 4 scallions
- ¼ cup almond flour
- 1 tsp sea salt
- ½ tsp garlic powder
- ¼ cup filtered water, as needed

Directions:

1. Place the zucchini, carrot, yellow squash, onion, scallions, almond flour, salt, and garlic powder in a food processor. Pulse until blended.
2. Add water to make the mixture moist, not runny. The batter will be fairly thick.
3. Spray a nonstick skillet or griddle with cooking spray and heat over medium-high heat.
4. Use an ice cream scoop or ¼-cup measure to drop the batter into the skillet. With a fork, spread the batter evenly, pressing down on the pancakes.
5. Cook, turning once, until browned on both sides, 5 minutes' total.
6. Serve hot or at room temperature.

Nutrition:

Carbohydrates – 33.4 g

Fiber – 7.2 g

Fat – 12.1 g

Protein – 6.3 g

Calories – 254

3. Tropical Granola

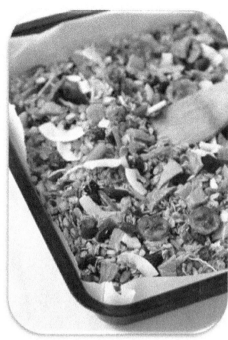

Preparation Time: 2 minutes

Cooking Time: 15 minutes

Servings: 4

Ingredients:

- 1 cup flaked unsweetened coconut
- 1 cup slivered almonds
- ½ cup flaxseed
- ½ cup raisins
- ½ tsp cinnamon
- ¼ tsp ginger
- ¼ tsp nutmeg
- ¼ tsp sea salt
- 1 vanilla bean, split lengthwise, deseeded
- ¼ cup coconut oil
- ½ cup unsweetened dried pineapple tidbits

Directions:

1. Preheat oven to 350° F.
2. In a medium bowl, combine the coconut, almonds, flaxseed, raisins, cinnamon, ginger, nutmeg, salt, vanilla bean seeds, and coconut oil. Mix until well combined.
3. Spread the mixture on a baking sheet and bake for 15 minutes, occasionally stirring, until golden brown.
4. Remove from the oven and cool, without stirring.
5. Once cooled, stir in the pineapple tidbits.
6. Store in an airtight container.

Nutrition:

Carbohydrates –44 g

Fiber – 3.8 g

Fat – 0.3 g

Protein – 2.3 g

Calories – 182

4. Summer Fruit Salad with Lime and Mint

Preparation Time: 10 minutes

Cooking Time: 0 minutes

Servings: 4

Ingredients:

- ¼ cup grapes
- ¼ cup peeled and diced apple
- ¼ cup bite-size watermelon pieces
- ¼ cup bite-size honeydew melon pieces
- ¼ cup bite-size cantaloupe pieces
- ¼ cup tangerine slices
- ¼ cup peeled and diced peaches
- ¼ cup strawberries
- 2 Tbsp chopped fresh mint
- 2 Tbsp freshly squeezed lemon juice

Directions:

1. In a medium bowl, combine all fruit.
2. Add the mint and lemon juice and mix well. Cover and refrigerate overnight.
3. Serve chilled.

Nutrition:

Carbohydrates – 7.8 g

Fiber – 0.09 g

Fat – 0.02 g

Protein – 0.6 g

Calories – 32

5. Winter Fruit Compote with Figs and Ginger

Preparation Time: 10 minutes

Cooking Time: 10 minutes

Servings: 4

Ingredients:

- 2 small tangerines, peeled, sectioned

- 1 apple, peeled, cored, diced
- ½ cup figs, stemmed and quartered
- ½ cup dried plums, halved
- ¼ cup dark cherries
- 1 cup filtered water
- 1 vanilla bean, split lengthwise, deseeded
- 1 tsp fresh ginger, grated
- ½ tsp cinnamon
- ½ tsp cloves
- 1 packet stevia (optional)

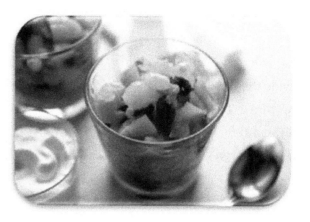

Directions:

1. In a medium saucepan, combine all ingredients.
2. Bring to a simmer over medium heat and cook, occasionally stirring, for 10 minutes, or until the fruit is tender but not too soft.
3. Remove from heat and let stand for 30 minutes.
4. Reheat if necessary and serve warm.

Nutrition:

Carbohydrates – 26 g

Fiber – 4.2 g

Fat – 0.4 g

Protein – 1 g

Calories – 102

6. All-American Apple Pie

Preparation Time: 10 minutes

Cooking Time: 10 minutes

Servings: 4

Ingredients:

- 4 apples, peeled, cored, sliced
- ½ cup orange juice, freshly squeezed
- 1 vanilla bean, cut lengthwise, deseeded
- ¼ tsp cinnamon
- ¼ cup unsweetened coconut milk

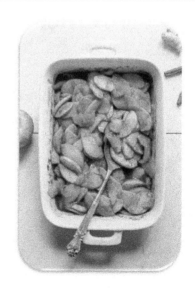

Directions:

1. In a bowl, combine all ingredients.
2. In a skillet set over medium heat, add the fruit mixture. Cook for 10 minutes.
3. Divide the mixture among four serving dishes and serve warm.
4. Top with 1 Tbsp coconut milk.

Nutrition:

Carbohydrates – 28.5 g

Fiber – 4.5 g

Fat – 0.1 g

Protein – 0.2 g

Calories – 109

7. Baby Potato Home Fries

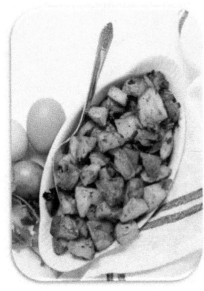

Preparation Time: 5 minutes

Cooking Time: 20 minutes

Servings: 2

Ingredients:

- 4 medium baby white potatoes
- ¼ cup vegetable broth
- ½ sweet white onion, chopped
- 1 red bell pepper, seeded, diced
- ½ cup mushrooms, sliced, any type
- 1 tsp sea salt
- 1 tsp garlic powder

Directions:

1. In a medium microwave-safe bowl, microwave the potatoes for 4 minutes, or until soft. Let cool.
2. In a large nonstick skillet set over medium heat, add the broth, onion, and red bell pepper. Sauté the vegetables for 5 minutes.
3. While the onion and peppers cook, cut the potatoes into quarters.
4. Add the potatoes, mushrooms, salt, and garlic powder to the skillet. Stir to combine. Cook for 10 minutes until the potatoes are crisp.
5. Serve warm.

Nutrition: Carbohydrates – 74.8 g

Fiber – 12.4 g

Fat – 0.8 g

Protein – 9.3 g

Calories – 337

8. Breakfast Fajitas

Preparation Time: 5 minutes

Cooking Time: 10 minutes

Servings: 2

Ingredients:

- 1 bell pepper, any color, seeded, sliced
- 1 sweet onion, chopped
- 1 cup cooked broccoli florets
- ½ cup mushrooms, sliced
- 1 cup cherry tomatoes, halved if large
- ½ cup sliced zucchini, or other squash
- 2 garlic cloves, peeled, chopped
- 1 jalapeño, chopped
- 1 tsp sea salt
- ½ tsp cumin
- 2 Tbsp fresh cilantro
- Juice of ½ lime

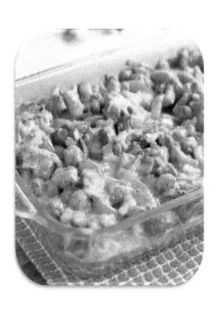

Directions:

1. Spray a nonstick skillet with cooking spray and place it over medium heat.
2. Add the bell pepper, onion, broccoli, mushrooms, tomatoes, zucchini, garlic, and jalapeño. Cook for 7 minutes, or until the desired level of tenderness, occasionally stirring.
3. Stir in the salt, cumin, and cilantro. Cook, stirring, for 3 minutes more.
4. Remove from heat and add the lime juice.
5. Divide between two plates and serve.

Nutrition:

Carbohydrates – 17.4 g

Fiber – 5.1 g

Fat – 0.07 g

Protein – 4.1 g

9. Brown Rice Porridge

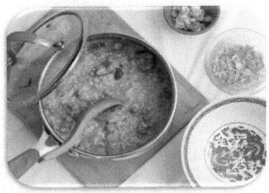

Preparation Time: 5 minutes

Cooking Time: 5 minutes

Servings: 6

Ingredients:

- 3 cups cooked brown rice
- 1 cup almond milk
- 1 packet stevia

Directions:

1. In a saucepan, combine the brown rice and the almond milk. Simmer over medium heat for 5 minutes, constantly stirring, until the mixture is thick and creamy.
2. Remove from heat and stir in the stevia.
3. Divide among 6 bowls and serve.

Nutrition:

Carbohydrates – 48.3 g

Fiber – 3.6 g

Fat – 1.8 g

Protein – 7 g

Calories – 236

10. Spaghetti Squash Hash Browns

Preparation Time: 2 minutes

Cooking Time: 10 minutes

Servings: 2

Ingredients:

- 2 cups cooked spaghetti squash
- ½ cup onion, finely chopped
- 1 tsp garlic powder
- ½ tsp sea salt

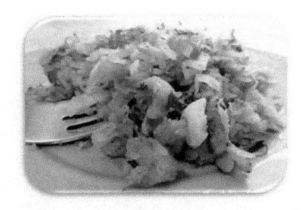

Directions:

1. Using paper towel, squeeze any excess moisture from the spaghetti squash.

Place the squash in a medium bowl. Add the onion, garlic powder, and salt. Mix to combine.

2. Spray a nonstick skillet with cooking spray and place it over medium heat.

3. Add the squash mixture to the pan. Cook, untouched, for 5 minutes. With a spatula, flip the hash browns. It's okay if the mixture falls apart. Cook for 5 minutes more until the desired level of crispness.

Nutrition:

Carbohydrates – 9.7 g

Fiber – 0.6 g

Fat – 0.6 g

Protein – 0.9 g

Calories – 44

11. Salad in Your Hand

Preparation Time: 10 minutes

Cooking Time: 0 minutes

Servings: 1

Ingredients:

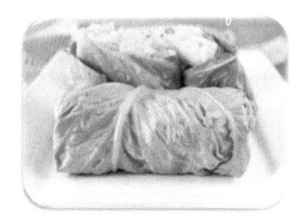

- 4 leaves lettuce, iceberg or romaine
- ½ avocado, diced
- 1 carrot, peeled, shredded
- ½ tomato, diced
- 1/3 cucumber, peeled, diced
- 1 Tbsp almonds, chopped

Directions:

1. Mix the avocado, carrot, cucumber, tomato, and almonds together.

2. Fill each leaf with one-quarter each of the mix and roll up.

Nutrition:

Carbohydrates – 17.8 g

Fiber – 6.5 g

Fat – 13.1 g

Protein – 4.1 g

Calories – 189

12. Warm Spinach Salad

Preparation Time: 2 minutes

Cooking Time: 5 minutes

Servings: 2

Ingredients:

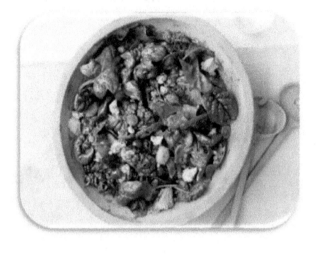

- 1 6-oz package baby spinach leaves
- ½ cup almonds, chopped, toasted
- 1 Tbsp sesame oil
- 1 Tbsp apple cider vinegar
- 1 tsp sea salt
- 1 cup shiitake mushrooms, chopped
- Water, as needed

Directions:

1. In a bowl, combine the spinach and almonds.
2. In a small saucepan over low heat, combine the sesame oil, cider vinegar, salt, and mushrooms. Cook for 5 minutes, adding water if it is absorbed.
3. Drizzle the mushroom dressing over the spinach and toss well to coat the spinach leaves.
4. Serve immediately.

Nutrition:

Carbohydrates – 20.3 g

Fiber – 7.6 g

Fat – 19.4 g

Protein – 10.2 g

Calories – 271

13. Salad on a Stick

Preparation Time: 5 minutes

Cooking Time: 0 minutes

Servings: 2

Ingredients:

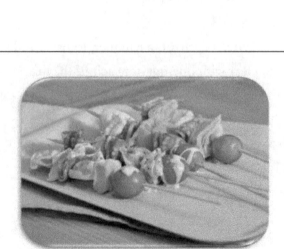

- 1 zucchini, sliced into 8 pieces
- 1 yellow squash, sliced into 8 pieces
- 1 cucumber, sliced into 8 pieces

- 8 cherry tomatoes
- 8 steamed broccoli florets
- 8 cauliflower florets
- 2 Tbsp blue cheese dressing

Directions:

1. On a wooden skewer, thread 1 zucchini slice, 1 yellow squash slice, 1 cucumber slice, 1 cherry tomato, 1 broccoli floret, and 1 cauliflower floret.
2. Repeat the process with remaining skewers and ingredients.
3. Drizzle with blue cheese dressing.

Nutrition:

Carbohydrates – 31.2 g

Fiber – 8.9 g

Fat – 1.5 g

Protein – 7.8 g

Calories – 142

14. Emeraland Forest Salad

Preparation Time: 5 minutes

Cooking Time: 0 minutes

Servings: 4

Ingredients:

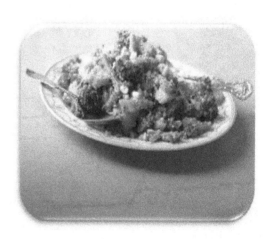

- 1 cup cooked broccoli florets, roughly chopped
- 1 cup asparagus spears, trimmed, cooked roughly chopped
- 2 cups cooked quinoa, cooled
- ½ cup water
- 2 Tbsp lemon juice, freshly squeezed
- 2 Tbsp coconut oil
- ½ tsp sea salt

Directions:

1. In a bowl, combine the broccoli and asparagus.
2. Stir in the quinoa.
3. In a blender, combine the water, lemon juice, coconut oil, and salt. Blend until the ingredients emulsify. Pour the dressing over the salad. Stir to combine.

4. Refrigerate the salad for 15 minutes to chill.

5. Serve cold.

Nutrition:

Carbohydrates – 53 g

Fiber – 6.2 g

Fat – 11.8 g

Protein – 12.2 g

Calories – 364

15. Summer Dinner Salad

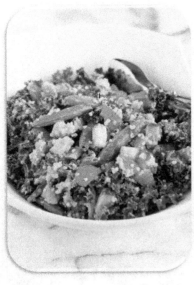

Preparation Time: 5 minutes

Cooking Time: 0 minutes

Servings: 4

Ingredients:

- 4 cups chopped iceberg or romaine lettuce
- 2 cups cherry tomatoes, halved
- 1 14.5-oz can whole green beans, drained
- ½ cup carrot, shredded
- 1 scallion, sliced
- 1 cucumber, peeled, sliced
- 2 radishes, thinly sliced

Directions:

1. In a bowl, combine all ingredients and toss with 2 Tbsp of your favorite dressing.

Nutrition:

Carbohydrates – 9 g

Fiber – 2.1 g

Fat – 0.3 g

Protein – 1.6 g

Calories – 39

16. Roasted Vegetable Salad

Preparation Time: 10 minutes

Cooking Time: 15 minutes

Servings: 2

Ingredients:

- 2 cups asparagus, chopped
- 1-pint cherry tomatoes
- ½ cup mushrooms halved
- 1 carrot, peeled, cut into bite-size pieces
- 1 red bell pepper, seeded, roughly chopped
- 1 Tbsp coconut oil
- 1 Tbsp garlic powder
- 1 tsp sea salt

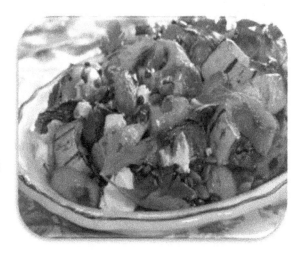

Directions:

1. Preheat the oven to 425°F.
2. In a bowl, combine all ingredients, coating the vegetables evenly.
3. Transfer the vegetables to a baking pan and roast for 15 minutes, or until the vegetables are tender.
4. Transfer the vegetables to a large bowl and serve either warm or cold.

Nutrition:

Carbohydrates – 15.4 g

Fiber – 4.2 g

Fat – 7.3 g

Protein – 2.9 g

Calories – 132

17. Quinoa and Avocado Salad

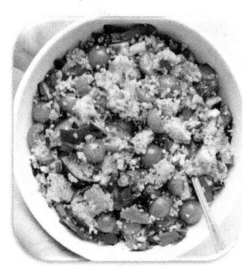

Preparation Time: 10 minutes

Cooking Time: 0 minutes

Servings: 2

Ingredients:

- 1 cup cooked quinoa, cooled
- 1 avocado, cut into cubes
- 5 oz fresh spinach, roughly chopped
- 1 cup cherry tomatoes, halved
- 1 cup cucumber, peeled, diced
- ¼ cup chopped cilantro
- 1 Tbsp garlic powder

- 1 Tbsp onion powder
- 1 tsp sea salt
- 1 Tbsp lemon juice, freshly squeezed

Directions:

1. In a bowl, combine all ingredients.
2. Chill for 15 minutes to allow the flavors to blend.
3. Serve immediately or keep refrigerated for 2 to 3 days.

Nutrition:

Carbohydrates – 63.6 g

Fiber – 9.9 g

Fat – 14.8 g

Protein – 13.7 g

Calories – 433

18.Avocado-Caprese Salad

Preparation Time: 5 minutes

Cooking Time: 0 minutes

Servings: 2

Ingredients:

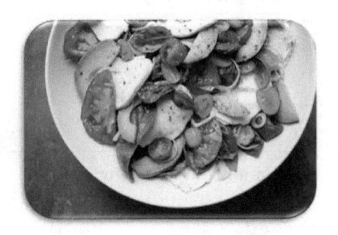

- 2 large heirloom tomatoes, sliced
- 1 avocado, sliced
- 1 bunch basil leaves
- 1 tsp sea salt

Directions:

1. In a bowl, toss all ingredients.
2. Season with the salt and serve.

Nutrition:

Carbohydrates – 9.1 g

Fiber – 4.9 g

Fat – 10.1 g

Protein – 2 g

Calories – 125

19. Spicy Sesame Noodle Salad

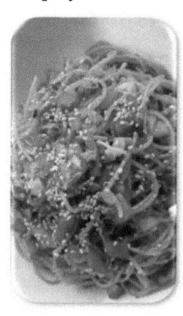

Preparation Time: 10 minutes

Cooking Time: 0 minutes

Servings: 4

Ingredients:

- 1 roasted spaghetti squash
- 2 cups cooked broccoli florets
- 1 bell pepper, seeded, cut into strips
- 1 scallion, chopped
- 1 Tbsp sesame oil
- 1 tsp red pepper flakes
- 1 tsp sea salt
- 2 Tbsp toasted sesame seeds

Directions:

1. Prepare the spaghetti squash "noodles" by removing the inside of the cooked squash with a fork into a large bowl.
2. Add the broccoli, red bell pepper, and scallion.
3. In a separate bowl, combine the sesame oil, red pepper flakes, and salt. Drizzle atop the vegetables. Toss gently to combine.
4. Garnish with the sesame seeds and serve.

Nutrition:

Carbohydrates – 6.4 g

Fiber – 2.5 g

Fat – 6 g

Protein – 2.5 g

Calories – 111

20. Organic Baby Tomato and Kale Salad

Preparation Time: 10 minutes

Cooking Time: 0 minutes

Servings: 2

Ingredients:

- 1 bunch kale, stemmed, leaves washed, chopped

- 2 cups organic baby tomatoes
- 2 tbsp Ranch Dressing

Directions:

1. In a bowl, combine all ingredients.
2. Divide equally onto two serving plates and enjoy immediately.

Nutrition:

Carbohydrates – 1.6 g

Fiber – 6.8 g

Fat – 6.9 g

Protein – 1.1 g

Calories – 58

21. The Asian Bowl

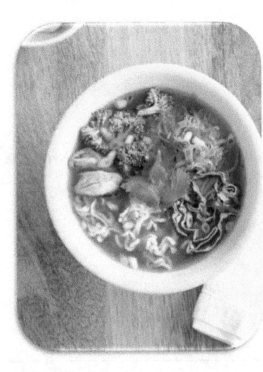

Preparation Time: 5 minutes

Cooking Time: 0 minutes

Servings: 1

Ingredients:

- 1 cup green cabbage, shredded
- 1 cup red cabbage, shredded
- 1 cup carrots, chopped
- ¼ cup water chestnuts
- 3 tbsp scallions, chopped
- 1 tbsp dark sesame oil
- 1 tbsp cashew butter
- ¼ tsp red pepper flakes, or additional as needed
- ½ tsp ginger powder
- Hot water, as needed
- 2 tsp toasted sesame seeds

Directions:

1. In a medium bowl, layer the green and red cabbage, then the carrots, water chestnuts, and scallions.
2. In a blender, add the sesame oil, cashew butter, red pepper flakes, and ginger powder. Blend until the ingredients emulsify. Add hot water by the teaspoon, if the dressing is too thick.
3. Pour the dressing over the vegetables, add sesame seeds, and serve.

Nutrition:

Carbohydrates – 20.8 g

Fiber – 6.6 g

Fat – 24.7 g

Protein – 7.2 g

Calories – 317

22. The Breakup Bowl

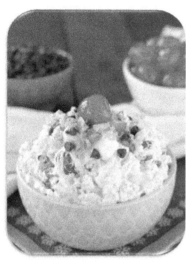

Preparation Time: 5 minutes

Cooking Time: 0 minutes

Servings: 1

Ingredients:

- 2 frozen bananas
- 2 Tbsp coconut milk
- 2 Tbsp fruit-sweetened-only strawberry jam
- 2 Tbsp unsweetened coconut, grated
- 2 Tbsp almonds, chopped, toasted
- ¼ cup coconut whipped cream

Directions:

1. In a food processor, combine bananas and coconut milk, blending until the mixture takes on the consistency of ice cream. Transfer to a single-serving bowl.
2. Top with the jam, coconut, toasted almonds, and whipped cream.
3. Serve immediately.

Nutrition:

Carbohydrates – 69.4 g

Fiber – 9.6 g

Fat – 19.2 g

Protein – 6.9 g

Calories – 454

23. The Fight It Off Bowl

Preparation Time: 5 minutes

Cooking Time: 10 minutes

Servings: 1

Ingredients:

- 2 cups vegetable broth
- 1 carrot, peeled, sliced
- ½ cup bite-size broccoli florets
- 2 garlic cloves, finely minced

Directions:

1. In a saucepan over medium heat, combine all ingredients. Cook for 10 minutes, or until vegetables reach a desired level of tenderness.
2. Pour into a bowl and eat.

Nutrition:

Carbohydrates – 12.8 g

Fiber – 2.8 g

Fat – 2.9 g

Protein – 11.8 g

Calories – 126

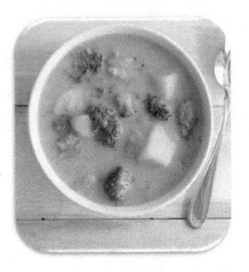

24. The Hawaiian Bowl

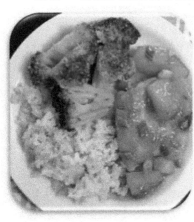

Preparation Time: 5 minutes

Cooking Time: 5 minutes

Servings: 1

Ingredients:

- ½ cup cooked brown rice
- 1 cup steamed broccoli
- ¼ cup packed-in-juice pineapple chunks, drained, liquid reserved
- 2 tbsp barbecue sauce

Directions:

1. In a medium bowl, layer the brown rice, broccoli, and pineapple.
2. In a saucepan over medium heat, whisk together the reserved pineapple juice and the barbecue sauce for 5 minutes, until thickened and bubbly.
3. Pour over the rice and broccoli and serve.

Nutrition:

Carbohydrates – 47.6 g

Fiber – 4.6 g

Fat – 1.6 g

Protein – 3.6 g

Calories – 223

25.   The Indian Bowl

Preparation Time: 10 minutes

Cooking Time: 5 minutes

Servings: 1

Ingredients:

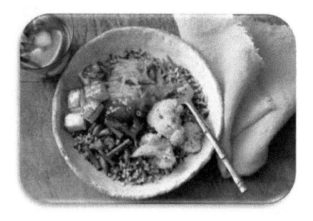

- 1 cup cooked quinoa, warmed
- 1 large carrot, peeled, sliced, steamed
- ½ cup cauliflower florets, cooked
- 1/8 cup chickpeas
- ¼ cup mushrooms, sliced
- ½ cup coconut milk
- 1 Tbsp yellow curry powder
- ½ tsp ground ginger
- 1 tsp sea salt
- 1 Tbsp tomato paste

Directions:

1. In a medium bowl, layer the quinoa, carrot, cauliflower, and chickpeas.
2. In a saucepan over medium heat, combine the mushrooms, coconut milk, curry powder, ginger, salt, and tomato paste. Whisk until the mixture simmers. Cook for 5 minutes and then let cool slightly.
3. Pour the sauce over the quinoa mixture and serve immediately.

Nutrition:

Carbohydrates – 26.1 g

Fiber – 13.5 g

Fat – 0.2 g

Protein – 5.4 g

Calories – 469

26. The Italian Bowl

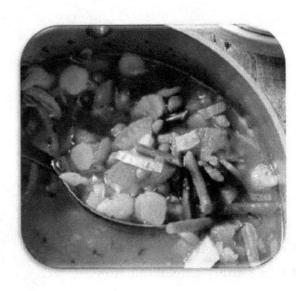

Preparation Time: 5 minutes

Cooking Time: 10 minutes

Servings: 1

Ingredients:

- 1 14.5-oz can tomatoes, whole, diced, or crushed, undrained
- 1 medium onion, diced
- ½ cup zucchini, sliced
- 4 garlic cloves, minced
- 1/3 cup fresh basil, chopped
- ½ tsp fresh oregano, chopped
- 2 Tbsp lemon juice, freshly squeezed
- 1 cup cooked quinoa, warmed
- ½ cup eggplant, peeled, diced, cooked, rewarmed

Directions:

1. Drain 2 tablespoons of liquid from the tomatoes and add it to a medium saucepan set over medium heat. Sir in the onion and sauté for 5 minutes, or until translucent.

2. Add the tomatoes with their remaining juices, zucchini, garlic, basil, and oregano. Stir to combine. Simmer for 5 minutes. Add the lemon juice.

3. In a single-serving bowl, layer the quinoa and the eggplant. Top with the tomato mixture.

4. Serve warm.

Nutrition:

Carbohydrates – 71.5 g

Fiber – 10.8 g

Fat – 5.4 g

Protein – 14.5 g

Calories – 390

27. The Mexican Bowl

Preparation Time: 10 minutes

Cooking Time: 0 minutes

Servings: 1

Ingredients:

- 1 cup sprouted black beans
- 1 tsp cumin, ground
- 1 medium sweet potato, cooked, diced
- 2/3 cup corn kernels
- ½ cup cilantro, chopped
- ½ avocado, diced
- 3 Tbsp salsa fresca
- Pinch sea salt

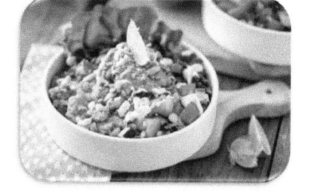

Directions:

1. In a small bowl, combine the beans, corn and the cumin.
2. In a medium microwaveable bowl, layer the sweet potatoes and top with the beans. Warm the vegetables in the microwave on high for 2 minutes, or until heated through.
3. Remove from the microwave and layer on the cilantro and avocado, and top with the salsa.
4. Season with salt and serve immediately.

Nutrition:

Carbohydrates – 69.5 g

Fiber – 17.4 g

Fat – 11.4 g

Protein – 17.8 g

Calories – 436

28. The Rose Bowl

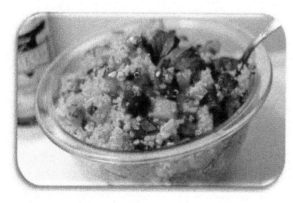

Preparation Time: 5 minutes

Cooking Time: 2 minutes

Servings: 1

Ingredients:

- 1 cup red quinoa, cooked
- ½ cup red peppers, roasted, diced
- ½ cup dark red cherries, pitted, sliced
- ¾ tsp red curry paste
- ½ cup coconut milk

Directions:

1. In a single-serving bowl, layer the quinoa, red peppers, and cherries.

2. In a blender, mix the curry paste and coconut milk. Pour the liquid over the layered quinoa, peppers, and cherries.

3. Microwave on high for 2 minutes.

Nutrition:

Carbohydrates – 64.5 g

Fiber – 6.7 g

Fat – 1.8 g

Protein – 16.7 g

Calories – 401

29. The Southern Bowl

Preparation Time: 5 minutes

Cooking Time: 50 minutes

Servings: 1

Ingredients:

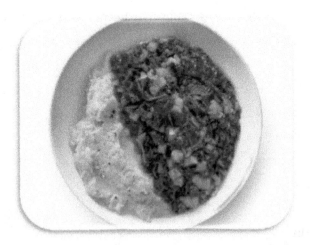

- ¼ cup vegetable broth, divided
- ¼ sweet onion, chopped
- 1 garlic clove, finely chopped
- ½ tsp sea salt, divided
- 4 ounces canned tomatoes, diced
- 1 cup collard greens
- 1 okra, fresh or frozen, sliced
- 1 sweet potato, peeled, cut into bite-size pieces
- ¼ cup almond milk

Directions:

1. In a saucepan over medium heat, heat 2 Tbsp vegetable broth. Add the onion and sauté for 5 minutes, or until translucent.

2. Add the garlic, ¼ tsp salt, tomatoes, the remaining 2 Tbsp broth, collard greens, and okra. Simmer for 30-35 minutes, or until tender.

3. In a pot of boiling water, cook the sweet potato pieces for 10 minutes, or until tender. Drain and place in a medium bowl.

4. To the potatoes, add the almond milk and remaining ¼ tsp salt. Using an electric mixer, mash the sweet potatoes.

5. Place the warm mashed sweet potato in a bowl. In another bowl, add the collard greens and okra mixture.

Nutrition:

Carbohydrates – 37.5 g

Fiber – 7.3 g

Fat – 2.7 g

Protein – 9 g

Calories – 201

30. Simple Bread

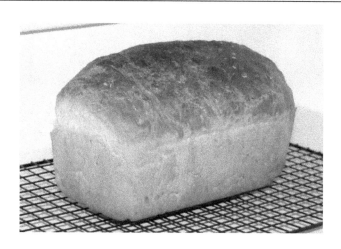

Preparation Time: 10 minutes

Cooking Time: 1 hour 10 minutes

Servings: 8 1-inch thick slices

Ingredients:

- 4 cups spelt flour
- 4 tablespoons sesame seeds
- 1 teaspoon baking soda
- ¼ teaspoon sea salt
- 10-12 drops liquid stevia
- 2 cups plus 2 tablespoons unsweetened almond milk

Directions:

1. Preheat oven to 350 degrees F. Line a 9x5-inch loaf pan with greased parchment paper.
2. In a large bowl, add all the ingredients and mix until well combined.
3. Transfer the mixture to the prepared loaf pan evenly.
4. Bake for 1 hour and 10 minutes or until a toothpick inserted in the center comes out clean.
5. Remove from oven and place the loaf pan onto a wire rack to cool for at least 10 minutes.
6. Carefully, invert the bread onto the rack to cool completely.
7. With a sharp knife, cut the bread loaf into desired sized slices and serve.

Nutrition:

Calories 239

Total Fat 4.2 g

Saturated Fat 0.6 g

Cholesterol 0 mg

Sodium 281 mg

Total Carbs 45.1 g

Fiber 8.1 g

Sugar 0.3 g

Protein 9.3 g

31.Banana Pancakes

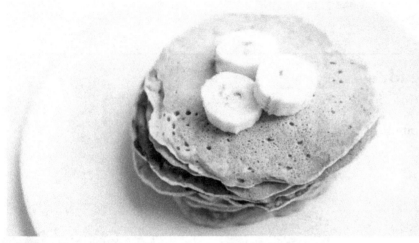

Preparation Time: 15 minutes

Cooking Time: 8 minutes

Servings: 2

Ingredients:

- ¼ cup rolled oats
- ¼ cup arrowroot flour
- ½ teaspoon organic baking powder
- ¼ teaspoon organic baking soda
- 1/8 teaspoon ground cinnamon
- ¼ cup unsweetened almond milk
- 2 organic egg whites
- 2 teaspoons almond butter
- ½ banana, peeled and mashed well
- 1/8 teaspoon organic vanilla extract
- 1 teaspoon olive oil
- ½ banana, peeled and sliced

Directions:

1. In a large bowl, add the flour, oats, baking soda, baking powder, and cinnamon and mix well.

2. In another bowl, add the almond milk, egg whites, almond butter, mashed banana, and vanilla and beat until well combined.
3. Add the flour mixture and mix until well combined.
4. In a large frying pan, heat the oil over medium-low heat.
5. Add half of the mixture and cook for about 1-2 minutes.
6. Flip to the other side and cook for 1-2 minutes more.
7. Repeat with the remaining mixture.
8. Serve topped with banana slices.

Nutrition:

Calories 244

Total Fat 12.7 g

Saturated Fat 1.3 g

Cholesterol 0 mg

Sodium 222 mg

Total Carbs 26.6 g

Fiber 4.6 g

Sugar 8.3 g

Protein 9.8 g

32. Refreshing Red Juice

Preparation Time: 10 minutes

Cooking Time: 0 minutes

Servings: 2

Ingredients:

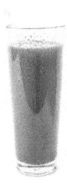

- 2 beets, peeled and roughly diced
- 1 large red bell pepper, seeded and chopped
- 1 large tomato, seeded and chopped
- 2 large red apples, cored and sliced
- 2½ cups fresh strawberries, hulled and sliced
- ¼ cup fresh mint leaves

Directions:

1. Add all ingredients to a juicer and extract the juice according to manufacturer's directions.
2. Transfer into two glasses and serve immediately.

Nutrition:

Calories 258

Total Fat 1.5 g

Saturated Fat 0.1 g

Cholesterol 0 mg

Sodium 90 mg

Total Carbs 63.6 g

Fiber 13.7 g

Sugar 45.4 g

Protein 5.3 g

33. Green Fruit Juice

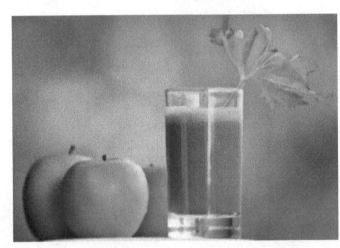

Preparation Time: 10 minutes

Cooking Time: 0 minutes

Servings: 2

Ingredients:

- 4 large kiwis, peeled and chopped
- 2 large green apples, cored and sliced
- 1 cup seedless green grapes
- 2 teaspoons lime juice

Directions:

1. Add all ingredients to a juicer and extract the juice according to manufacturer's directions.
2. Transfer into two glasses and serve immediately.

Nutrition:

Calories 240

Total Fat 1.4 g

Saturated Fat 0.1 g

Cholesterol 0 mg

Sodium 7 mg

Total Carbs 61 g

Fiber 10.4 g

Sugar 44.3 g

Protein 2.6 g

34. Bell Pepper and Mushroom Omelet

Preparation Time: 15 minutes

Cooking Time: 25 minutes

Servings: 4

Ingredients:

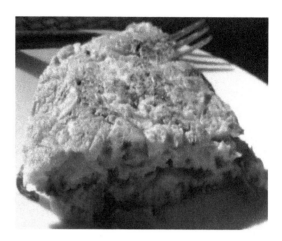

- 6 large organic eggs
- Sea salt and freshly ground black pepper, to taste
- ½ cup unsweetened almond milk
- ½ of an onion, chopped
- ¼ cup fresh mushrooms, cut into slices
- ¼ cup red bell pepper, seeded and diced
- 1 tablespoon chives, minced

Directions:

1. Preheat the oven to 350 degrees F. Lightly grease a pie dish.
2. In a bowl, add the eggs, salt, black pepper, and almond milk and beat until well combined.
3. In another bowl, mix together the onion, bell pepper, and mushrooms.
4. Transfer the egg mixture into the prepared pie dish evenly.
5. Top with vegetable mixture evenly.
6. Sprinkle with chives evenly.
7. Bake for about 20-25 minutes.
8. With a knife, cut into equal sized wedges and serve.

Nutrition:

Calories 121

Total Fat 8 g

Saturated Fat 2.4 g

Cholesterol 279 mg

Sodium 187 mg

Total Carbs 2.9 g

Fiber 0.6 g

Sugar 1.6 g

Protein 10 g

35. Tofu and Veggie Scramble

Preparation Time: 15 minutes

Cooking Time: 15 minutes

Servings: 2

Ingredients:

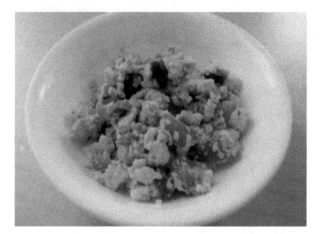

- ½ tablespoon olive oil
- 1 small onion, chopped finely
- 1 small red bell pepper, seeded and chopped finely
- 1 cup cherry tomatoes, chopped finely
- 1½ cups firm tofu, crumbled and chopped
- Pinch of cayenne pepper
- Pinch of ground turmeric
- Sea salt, to taste

Directions:

1. In a skillet, heat oil over medium heat and sauté the onion and bell pepper for about 4-5 minute.
2. Add the tomatoes and cook for about 1-2 minutes.
3. Add the tofu, turmeric, cayenne pepper and salt and cook for about 6-8 minutes.
4. Serve hot.

Nutrition: Calories 212

Total Fat 11.8 g; Saturated Fat 2.2 g;

Cholesterol 0 mg; Sodium 147 mg; Total Carbs 14.6 g

Fiber 4.4 g; Sugar 8 g; Protein 17.3 g

36. Apple Porridge

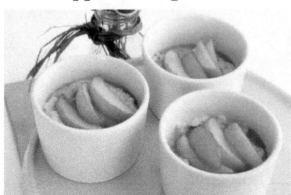

Preparation Time: 10 minutes

Cooking Time: 5 minutes

Servings: 4

Ingredients:

- 2 cups unsweetened almond milk
- 3 tablespoons walnuts, chopped
- 3 tablespoons sunflower seeds
- 2 large apples, peeled, cored, and grated

- ½ teaspoon organic vanilla extract
- Pinch of ground cinnamon
- ½ small apple, cored and sliced

Directions:

1. In a large pan, mix together the milk, walnuts, sunflower seeds, grated apple, vanilla, and cinnamon over medium-low heat and cook for about 3-5 minutes.
2. Remove from the heat and transfer the porridge into serving bowls.
3. Top with remaining apple slices and serve.

Nutrition:

Calories 143

Total Fat 6.6 g

Saturated Fat 0.5 g

Cholesterol 0 mg

Sodium 92 mg

Total Carbs 21.4 g

Fiber 4.5 g

Sugar 14.7 g

Protein 2.7 g

37. Overnight Chocolate Oatmeal

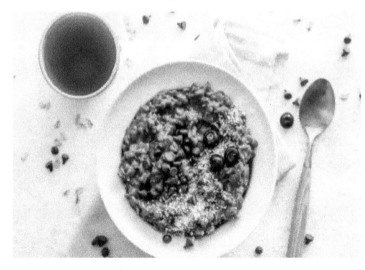

Preparation Time: 10 minutes

Cooking Time: 0 minutes

Servings: 2

Ingredients:

- 1 cup unsweetened almond milk
- 1 cup rolled oats
- 1 tablespoon cacao powder
- 8-10 drops liquid stevia
- ¼ cup fresh blueberries
- 1 tablespoon unsweetened dark mini chocolate chips

Directions:

1. In a large bowl, add all the ingredients except blueberries and chocolate chips and mix until well combined.

2. Cover the bowl and refrigerate overnight.

3. Top with chocolate chips and blueberries and serve.

Nutrition:

Calories 209

Total Fat 6 g

Saturated Fat 1.5 g

Cholesterol 0 mg

Sodium 93 mg

Total Carbs 35.1 g

Fiber 5.8 g

Sugar 4.2 g

Protein 6.8 g

38. Zucchini Bread

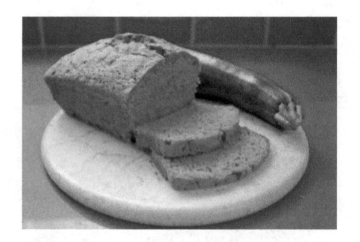

Preparation Time: 15 minutes

Cooking Time: 45 minutes

Servings: 6 1-inch thick slices

Ingredients:

- ½ cup almond flour, sifted
- 1½ teaspoons baking soda
- ½ teaspoon ground cinnamon
- ¼ teaspoon ground cardamom
- 1½ cups banana, peeled and mashed
- ¼ cup almond butter, softened
- 2 teaspoons organic vanilla extract
- 1 cup zucchini, shredded

Directions:

1. Preheat oven to 350 degrees F. Grease a 6x3-inch loaf pan.

2. In a large bowl, mix the flour, baking soda, and spices.

3. In another bowl, add the remaining ingredients except zucchini and beat until well combined.

4. Add the flour mixture and mix until just combined.

5. Fold in the grated zucchini.

6. Transfer the batter into the prepared loaf pan.

7. Bake for about 40-45 minutes or until a toothpick inserted in the center comes out clean.
8. Remove from oven and place the loaf pan onto a wire rack to cool for at least 10 minutes.
9. Carefully, invert the bread onto the rack to cool completely before slicing.
10. With a sharp knife, cut the bread loaf into 6 equal sized slices and serve.

Nutrition:

Calories 161

Total Fat 10.5 g

Saturated Fat 1.5 g

Cholesterol 0 mg

Sodium 319 mg

Total Carbs 14.7 g

Fiber 2.6 g

Sugar 5.5 g

Protein 4.7 g

39. Vanilla Waffles

Preparation Time: 10 minutes

Cooking Time: 10 minutes

Servings: 2

Ingredients:

- ¼ cup coconut flour
- 1 teaspoon baking powder
- 6 organic egg whites
- ¼ cup unsweetened almond milk
- 1 tablespoon agave syrup
- 1/8 teaspoon organic vanilla extract
- 4-6 fresh strawberries, hulled and sliced

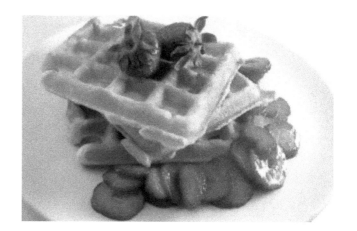

Directions:

1. Preheat the waffle iron and lightly grease it.
2. In a large bowl, add the flour and baking powder and mix well.
3. Add the remaining ingredients except the strawberries and mix until well combined.
4. Place half of the mixture to the preheated waffle iron.
5. Cook for about 3-5 minutes or until waffles become golden brown.

6. Repeat with the remaining mixture.
7. Serve warm topped with the strawberry slices.

Nutrition:

Calories 107

Total Fat 0.9 g

Saturated Fat 0.3 g

Cholesterol 0 mg

Sodium 136 mg

Total Carbs 13.4 g

Fiber 1.3 g

Sugar 2 g

Protein 11.3 g

Lunch Recipes

40. Chicken-Sausage Frittata with Corn And Feta Recipe

Preparation Time: 15 minutes

Cooking Time: 10 minutes

Servings: serves 4

Ingredients:

- 2 tablespoons extra-virgin olive oil
- 3 links chicken sausage, cut into quarters
- 1 small onion, diced
- 8 large eggs
- Kosher salt and freshly ground black pepper
- ½ cup crumbled feta, preferably Bulgarian
- 1 jalapeño, diced
- 1 yellow bell pepper, diced
- 1 orange bell pepper, diced
- 1 ripe avocado, diced
- ½ cup cilantro leaves
- 1 ear of corn then kernels cut off the cob

Directions:

1. Adjust the broiler rack from the heat source to 10 inches, and preheat the broiler to high. Beat the eggs with 2 generous pinches of salt and the feta in a wide pot. Deposit aside.

2. Heat oil over medium - high heat in a 12-inch skillet, until shimmering. Attach the onion and cook, stirring for about 2 minutes, until softened. Top with pepper and salt. Stir in jalapeño, bell peppers, corn and chicken sausage and cook for about 6 minutes until browned.

3. Attach the eggs and cook, stirring, for 1 to 2 minutes until moist curds have formed. Switch to broiler and cook for around 3 minutes, until the top is set. Allow the frittata to cool a bit, then use a spatula to loosen the bottom and sides. Flip out the frittata carefully using a plate larger than the saucepan. Cut into wedges and serve with a sliced cilantro and avocado.

Nutrition:

Calories: 240

Carbohydrates: 4 grams

Fat: 18 grams

Protein: 17 grams

41. Alkaline Cauliflower Fried Rice

Preparation Time: 5 min

Cooking Time: 5 min

Servings: 4

Ingredients:

- 1 zucchini (courgette)
- 1 inch fresh root ginger
- 1 inch fresh root turmeric
- 1 large cauliflower
- 1/2 bunch of kale (any variety)
- 1 tbsp coconut oil
- 1 bunch of coriander
- 1/2 bunch parsley (any variety)
- 1 bunch mint
- 1 tbsp tamari soy sauce or Bragg liquid aminos
- 1 lime
- 4 spring onions
- 2 handfuls almonds
- Optional
- 1 green chili
- Instead of ginger and fresh turmeric, use 1 teaspoon of each powdered

Directions:

1. Begin by making the rice of cauliflower–it's very easy–just split the cauliflower into small florets and chop it into your blender or food processor and pulse until it's like rice. Unless you don't have the blender, you can only grate it and get an effect that is very close.

2. Now is veggie preparation time, so thinly slice your kale, quarter and then thinly slice the courgette (zucchini) and chop all your herbs roughly next, prepare your ginger and turmeric–first by peeling them (for quick peeling, just scrape back of a spoon over the ginger / turmeric–sweet!) And then rub them in a big.

3. Stir the coriander into the mix including the stems as this begins warming up.

4. Stir in the cauliflower after 30 seconds and then the kale after another 2 min-3 minutes, add the spring onions and then the rest of the herbs, the Bragg/tamari and stir through–and then remove from the heat–the total cooking time will be less than 5 minutes–you don't want it to go too soft!

5. Now chop and mix the almonds roughly, season to taste and add lime juice according to your favorite.

Nutrition:

Calories: 109.5

Fat: 7.5 grams

Cholesterol: 93.5 grams

Carbohydrates: 6.8 grams

Protein: 5.3 grams

42. Creamy Avocado Cilantro Lime Dressing Recipe

Preparation Time: 20 minutes

Cooking Time: 10 minutes

Servings: 6-8

Ingredients:

- ¼ cup olive oil
- ¼ teaspoon sea salt
- ½ cup cilantro, chopped
- ¼ cup plain goat yogurt
- Juice of ½ lime
- 1 teaspoon lime zest
- 1 avocado
- 1 clove garlic, peeled
- ½ jalapeno, chopped
- ¼ teaspoon pepper
- ½ teaspoon cumin

Directions:

1. Place/put all the ingredients in a food processor or mixer and mix until well balanced.

Nutrition:

123 calories

1-gram protein

12 grams fat

3.6 grams carbohydrate

0.8 grams sugar

43. Creamy Avocado Dressing

Preparation Time: 5 min

Cooking Time: 5 min

Servings: 4

Ingredients:

- 1/4 teaspoon ground black pepper
- Water, as needed
- 1 whole large avocado
- 1 clove garlic, peeled
- 1/2 tbspoon fresh lime or lemon juice
- 3 tablespoons olive oil or avocado oil
- 1/4 teaspoon kosher salt

Directions:

1. Put the peeled clove of garlic, lime or lemon juice, avocado, olive oil, salt and pepper into a mini food processor.
2. Process till smooth, stopping a few times to scrape the sides down. Thin the salad dressing out with some water (1/4 cup to 1/2 cup) before a perfect consistency is achieved.
3. Maintain/keep at least a week in an airtight container, but 3 to 4 days is best.

Nutrition:

Calories: 38.2

Total fat: 2.6 grams

Saturated fat: 0.6 grams

Cholesterol: 1.2 milligrams

Sodium: 8.8 milligrams

Potassium: 76.9 milligrams

Total carbohydrate: 3.6 grams

Dietary fiber: 1.0 grams

Sugars: 0.9 grams

44.Southwestern Avocado Salad Dressing

Preparation Time: 5 minutes

Cooking Time: 1 hour

Servings: 8

Ingredients:

- 1 ripe avocado
- 1 cup buttermilk
- 1/2 teaspoon garlic powder
- 1/2 teaspoon chipotle chili powder
- 1/2 teaspoon salt
- 1/4 cup cilantro
- Juice of 1/2 lime
- 1 teaspoon ranch seasoning powder homemade or store bought

Directions:

1. Break the avocado in half, extract the pit from the flesh and scoop the skin.
2. Attach all the other ingredients to a mixer.
3. Blend in until creamy and smooth.
4. Before serving, refrigerate for one hour.
5. Keeps in the refrigerator for 3 days.

Nutrition:

Calories: 61

Calories from fat: 36

Total fat: 4 grams

Saturated fat: 1 gram

Cholesterol: 3 milligrams

Sodium: 237 milligrams

Potassium: 162 milligrams

Total carbohydrates: 4 grams

Dietary fiber: 1 gram

Sugars: 1 gram

Protein: 1 gram

45. Brain Boosting Smoothie Recipe

Preparation Time: 5 minutes

Cooking Time: 5 minutes

Servings: 1

Ingredients:

- ½ avocado

- ½ banana
- ½ cup blueberries
- 6 walnuts
- 1 scoop vanilla whey protein powder
- ½ cup water

Directions:

1. Add/put all ingredients to blender then blend until smooth texture is reached.

Nutrition:

Calories: 400

Fat: 13grams

Protein: 7grams

Carbohydrates: 68grams

Fiber: 10grams

Sugar: 50grams

46.Lemon Avocado Salad Dressing

Preparation Time: 5 minutes

Cooking Time: 5 minutes

Servings: 2-3

Ingredients:

- 2 tablespoons olive oil
- 1 garlic clove, minced
- 1/2 teaspoon seasoned salt
- 1 medium ripe avocado, peeled and mashed
- 1/4 cup water
- 2 tablespoons sour cream
- 2 tablespoons lemon juice
- 1 tbspoon minced fresh dill or 1 teaspoon dill weed
- 1/2 teaspoon honey
- Salad greens, cherry tomatoes, sliced cucumbers and sweet red and yellow pepper strips

Directions:

1. In a blender, combine the first nine ingredients; cover and process until blended.
2. Serve with salad greens, tomatoes, cucumbers and peppers. Store in the refrigerator.

Nutrition:

Calories: 38.2

Total fat: 2.6 grams

Saturated fat: 0.6 grams

Cholesterol: 1.2 milligrams

Sodium: 8.8 milligrams

Potassium: 76.9 milligrams

Total carbohydrate: 3.6 grams

Dietary fiber: 1.0 grams

Sugars: 0.9 grams

Protein: 0.8 grams

47.Avocado Salad With Bell Pepper And Tomatoes

Preparation Time: 5 minutes

Cooking Time: 5 minutes

Servings: 2-3

Ingredients:

- Coarse salt
- 1 firm, ripe avocado, halved and pitted
- 6 cherry tomatoes, halved
- 1 teaspoon extra-virgin olive oil
- Juice of 1/2 lime
- 1 scallion, trimmed and thinly sliced
- 1 tbspoon chopped fresh cilantro leaves, with whole leaves for garnish
- 1 small garlic clove, minced
- Pinch of cayenne pepper
- 1/2 yellow bell pepper, ribs and seeds removed, diced

Directions:

1. Whisk the olive oil, lime juice, garlic, and cayenne together in a small bowl. Season with the salt.
2. From the avocado halves, scoop out flesh, conserve shells and chop. Switch to a bowl and add chopped cilantro, bell pepper, onions, scallion.
3. Drizzle with salt and season with dressing. Stir gently to mix. Mix spoon into allocated containers. Garnish with whole leaves of cilantro and serve right away.

Nutrition:

Calories: 424

Fiber: 16.36 grams

Saturated fat: 5 grams

Carbohydrates: 31.25 grams

Fat 34.63: grams

Protein 6.6: grams

48.Avocado Egg Salad

Preparation Time: 10 minutes

Cooking Time: 5 minutes

Servings: 4

Ingredients:

- 2 eggs, hard boiled
- 1 avocado, finely chopped
- 3 tablespoons boiled corn
- 1 tomato, thinly chopped
- 1 tablespoon extra-virgin olive oil
- Salt to taste
- 1 tablespoon lemon juice
- 3 green onions, chopped

Directions:

1. In a large bowl, whisk in chopped avocado and lemon juice.
2. In the same bowl, mix it with other ingredients, except for tomato.
3. Serve on slices of bread with sliced tomatoes.

Nutrition:

Calories: 119

Fat: 8.7 g

Cholesterol: 125 mg

Carbohydrates: 3.4 g

Protein: 7.2 g

49.Avocado Caprese Salad

Preparation Time: 5 minutes

Cooking Time: 5 minutes

Servings: 1

Ingredients:

- 1 1/2 teaspoons balsamic vinegar
- Generous pinch of sugar/dollop of honey
- 3 slices fresh mozzarella cheese
- Fresh basil leaves
- 2 cups fresh arugula
- 2-3 Campari or cocktail style tomatoes sliced
- 1/2 avocado pitted and sliced
- 1 tablespoon extra-virgin olive oil
- Kosher salt and freshly ground black pepper

Directions:

1. In a serving bowl, add the arugula, onion, avocado slices, and mozzarella.
2. Fill with leaves of broken or slivered basil.
3. With the balsamic vinegar, sugar or honey, whisk the extra virgin olive oil in a small bowl and season with kosher salt and freshly ground black pepper to taste and pour over the salad.
4. Throw coat and serve.

Nutrition:

Calories: 164.2

Fat: 11.8 grams

Cholesterol: 10.0 milligrams

Carbohydrates: 11.6 grams

Fiber: 4.7 grams

Sugar: 5 grams

Protein: 5.4 grams

50.Avocado Salmon Salad With Arugula

Preparation Time: 10 minutes

Cooking Time: 5 minutes

Servings: 1

Ingredients:

- 2 green onions, sliced thinly
- 8 cherry tomatoes, halved (or a mix of yellow and red)
- ¾ pound salmon fillet
- 1 avocado, pitted, peeled and chopped

- 1 small (raw) zucchini, thinly sliced in half moons
- 4 radishes, thinly sliced
- 1 recipe avocado citrus dressing

Directions:

1. Preheat to 400 ° f on oven. Line a small saucepan with parchment paper.
2. Arrange salmon on the pan, skin down, and bake for 10 to 12 minutes until just cooked.
3. Warm slightly, cut fat, flake flesh and set aside.
4. Divide arugula between serving plates. Top with salmon and avocado, courgettes, red onion and tomatoes.
5. Serve in citrus dressing with creamy avocado

Nutrition:

Calories: 320

Fat: 32 grams

Cholesterol: 5 milligrams

Potassium: 210 milligrams

Carbohydrates: 6 grams

Fiber: 3 grams

Protein: 6 grams

51.Alkaline Spaghetti Squash Recipe

Preparation Time: 10 minutes

Cooking Time: 30 minutes

Servings: 4

Ingredients:

- 1 spaghetti squash
- Grapeseed oil
- Sea salt
- Cayenne powder (optional)
- Onion powder (optional)

Directions:

1. Preheat your oven to 375°f
2. Carefully chop off the ends of the squash and cut it in half.
3. Scoop out the seeds into a bowl.
4. Coat the squash with oil.

5. Season the squash and flip it over for the other side to get baked. When properly baked, the outside of the squash will be tender.

6. Allow the squash to cool off, then, use a fork to scrape the inside into a bowl.

7. Add seasoning to taste.

8. Dish your alkaline spaghetti squash!

Nutrition:

Calories: 672

Carbohydrates: 65 grams

Fat: 47 grams

Protein: 12 grams

52. Tomato and Greens Salad

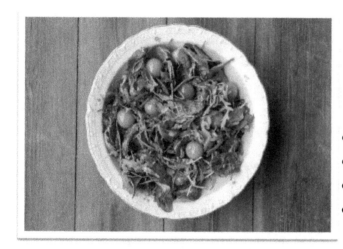

Preparation Time: 10 minutes

Cooking Time: 10 minutes

Servings: 4

Ingredients:

- 6 cups fresh baby greens
- 3 cups cherry tomatoes
- 2 tablespoons extra-virgin olive oil
- 1 tablespoon fresh lemon juice

Directions:

1. In a large bowl, add all ingredients and toss to coat well.

2. Serve immediately.

Nutrition:

Calories 90; Total Fat 7.3 g; Saturated Fat 1.1 g

Cholesterol 0 mg; Sodium 12 mg; Total Carbs 6.3 g

Fiber 2.2 g; Sugar 4.2 g; Protein 1.7 g

53. Cucumber and Onion Salad

Preparation Time: 10 minutes

Cooking Time: 0 minutes

Servings: 5

Ingredients:

- 3 large cucumbers, sliced thinly
- ½ cup onion, sliced
- 2 tablespoons olive oil
- 1 tablespoon fresh apple cider vinegar
- Sea salt, to taste
- ¼ cup fresh cilantro, chopped

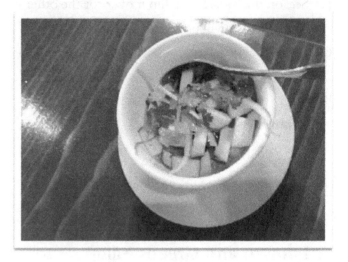

Directions:

1. In a large bowl, add all ingredients and toss to coat well.
2. Serve immediately.

Nutrition:

Calories 81; Total Fat 5.8 g; Saturated Fat 0.9g

Cholesterol 0 mg; Sodium 49 mg; Total Carbs 7.7 g

Fiber 1.2 g; Sugar 3.5 g; Protein 1.3 g

54.Apple Salad

Preparation Time: 10 minutes

Cooking Time: 0 minutes

Servings: 4

Ingredients:

- 4 large apples, cored and sliced
- 6 cups fresh baby spinach
- 3 tablespoons extra-virgin olive oil
- 2 tablespoons apple cider vinegar

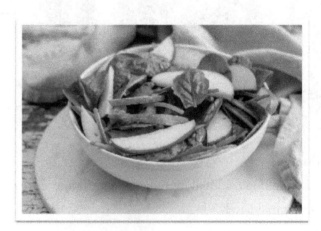

Directions:

1. In a large bowl, add all the ingredients and toss to coat well.
2. Serve immediately.

Nutrition:

Calories 218

Total Fat 11.1 g

Saturated Fat 1.5 g

Cholesterol 0 mg

Sodium 38 mg

Total Carbs 32.5 g

Fiber 6.4 g

Sugar 23.4 g

Protein 1.9 g

55.Cauliflower Soup

Preparation Time: 10 minutes

Cooking Time: 25 minutes

Servings: 4

Ingredients:

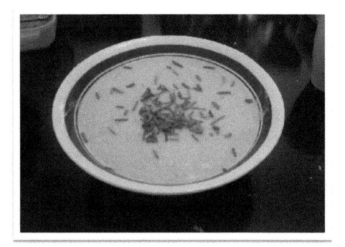

- 2 tablespoons olive oil
- 1 yellow onion, chopped
- 2 carrots, peeled and chopped
- 2 celery stalks, chopped
- 2 garlic cloves, minced
- 1 Serrano pepper, chopped finely
- 1 teaspoon ground turmeric
- 1 teaspoon ground coriander
- 1 teaspoon ground cumin
- ¼ teaspoon red pepper flakes, crushed
- 1 head cauliflower, chopped
- 4 cups vegetable broth
- 1 cup coconut milk
- Sea salt and freshly ground black pepper, to taste
- 2 tablespoons fresh chives, chopped

Directions:

1. In a large sauce pan, heat the oil over medium heat and sauté the onion, carrot, and celery for 5-6 minutes.
2. Add the garlic, Serrano pepper and spices and sauté for about 1 minute.
3. Add the cauliflower and cook for 5 minutes, stirring occasionally.
4. Add the broth and coconut milk and bring to a boil over medium-high heat.
5. Reduce the heat to low and simmer for 15 minutes.
6. Season the soup with salt and black pepper and remove from the heat.
7. Serve hot with a topping of chives.

Nutrition:

Calories 285; Total Fat 23 g; Saturated Fat 14.1 g

Cholesterol 0 mg; Sodium 861 mg; Total Carbs 14.9 g

Fiber 4.8 g; Sugar 7.2 g; Protein 8.5 g

56. Tomato Soup

Preparation Time: 10 minutes

Cooking Time: 45 minutes

Servings: 4

Ingredients:

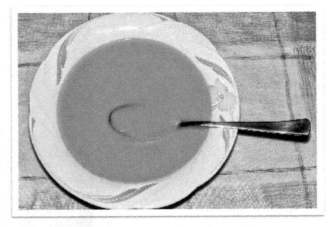

- 2 tablespoons coconut oil
- 2 carrots, peeled and chopped roughly
- 1 large white onion, chopped roughly
- 3 garlic cloves, minced
- 5 large tomatoes, chopped roughly
- ¼ cup fresh basil, chopped
- 1 tablespoon tomato paste
- 3 cups homemade vegetable broth
- ¼ cup coconut milk
- Sea salt and freshly ground black pepper, to taste

Directions:

1. In a large pan, melt the coconut oil over medium heat and cook the carrot and onion for about 10 minutes, stirring frequently.
2. Add the garlic and cook for 1-2 minutes.
3. Stir in the tomatoes, basil, tomato paste, and broth and bring to a boil.
4. Reduce the heat to low and simmer for about 30 minutes.
5. Stir in the coconut milk, salt, and black pepper and remove from the heat.
6. With an immersion blender, blend the soup until smooth.
7. Serve hot.

Nutrition:

Calories 197

Total Fat 12 g

Saturated Fat 9.4 g

Cholesterol 0 mg

Sodium 671 mg

Total Carbs 18.4 g

Fiber 4.8 g

Sugar 10.6 g

Protein 7 g

57.Asparagus Soup

Nutrition:

Calories 125; Total Fat 6.9 g; Saturated Fat 2.6 g

Cholesterol 0 mg; Sodium 510 mg; Total Carbs 8.9 g

Fiber 4.1 g; Sugar 4.6 g; Protein 9 g

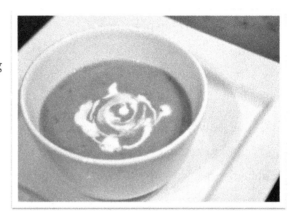

Preparation Time: 15 minutes

Cooking Time: 40 minutes

Servings: 4

Ingredients:

- 1 tablespoon olive oil
- 3 scallions, chopped
- 1½ pounds fresh asparagus, trimmed and chopped
- 4 cups homemade vegetable broth
- 2 tablespoons freshly squeezed lemon juice
- Sea salt and freshly ground black pepper, to taste
- 2 tablespoons coconut cream

Directions:

1. In a large pan, heat the oil over medium heat and sauté the scallion for 4-5 minutes.
2. Stir in the asparagus and broth and bring to a boil.
3. Reduce the heat to low and simmer, covered for 25-30 minutes.
4. Remove from the heat and set aside to cool slightly.
5. Now, transfer the soup into a high-speed blender in 2 batches and pulse until smooth.
6. Return the soup into the same pan over medium heat and simmer for 4-5 minutes.
7. Stir in the lemon juice, salt, and black pepper and remove from the heat.
8. Serve hot with a topping of coconut cream.

58.Okra Curry

Preparation Time: 15 minutes

Cooking Time: 13 minutes

Servings: 2

Ingredients:

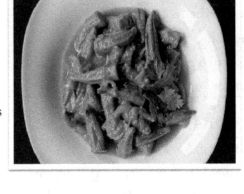

- 1 tablespoon olive oil
- ½ teaspoon cumin seeds
- ¾ pound okra pods, trimmed and cut into 2-inch pieces
- ½ teaspoon curry powder
- ½ teaspoon red chili powder
- 1 teaspoon ground coriander
- Sea salt and freshly ground black pepper, to taste

Directions:

1. In a large skillet, heat the oil over medium heat and sauté the cumin seeds for 30 seconds.
2. Add the okra and stir fry for 1-1½ minutes.
3. Reduce the heat to low and cook, covered for 6-8 minutes, stirring occasionally.
4. Uncover and increase the heat to medium.
5. Stir in curry powder, red chili powder, and coriander and cook for 2-3 more minutes.
6. Season with salt and remove from heat.
7. Serve hot.

Nutrition:

Calories 134; Total Fat 7.6 g; Saturated Fat 1.1 g

Cholesterol 0 mg; Sodium 137 mg; Total Carbs 13.6 g

Fiber 5.9 g; Sugar 2.6 g; Protein 3.5 g

59.Eggplant Curry

Preparation Time: 15 minutes

Cooking Time: 35 minutes

Servings: 3

Ingredients:

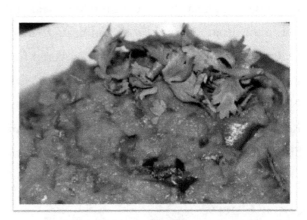

- 1 tablespoon coconut oil
- 1 medium onion, chopped finely
- 2 garlic cloves, minced
- ½ tablespoon fresh ginger, minced
- 1 Serrano pepper, seeded and minced
- 1 teaspoon curry powder

- ¼ teaspoon cayenne pepper
- Sea salt, to taste
- 1 medium tomato, finely chopped
- 1 large eggplant, cubed
- 1 cup unsweetened coconut milk
- 2 tablespoons fresh cilantro, chopped

Directions:

1. In a large skillet, melt the coconut oil over medium heat and sauté the onion for 8-9 minutes.
2. Add the garlic, garlic, Serrano pepper, curry powder, cayenne pepper, and salt and sauté for 1 minute.
3. Add the tomato and cook for 3-4 minutes, crushing with the back of spoon.
4. Add the eggplant and salt and cook for 1 minute, stirring occasionally.
5. Stir in the coconut milk and bring to a gentle boil.
6. Reduce the heat to medium-low and simmer, covered for 15-20 minutes or until done completely.
7. Serve with a garnish of cilantro.

Nutrition:

Calories 124

Total Fat 6.4 g

Saturated Fat 5.3 g

Cholesterol 0 mg

Sodium 86 mg

Total Carbs 16.6 g

Fiber 7.5 g

Sugar 7.4 g

Protein 2.6 g

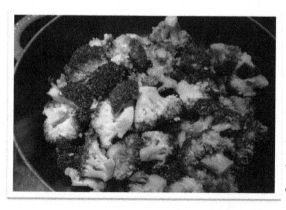

60. Garlicky Broccoli

Preparation Time: 10 minutes

Cooking Time: 8 minutes

Servings: 2

Ingredients:

- 1 tablespoon olive oil
- 2 garlic cloves, minced
- 2 cups broccoli florets

- 2 tablespoons water
- Sea salt and freshly ground black pepper, to taste

Directions:

1. In a large skillet, heat the oil over medium heat and sauté the garlic for about 1 minute.
2. Add the broccoli and stir fry for 2 minutes.
3. Stir in water, salt, and black pepper and stir fry for 4-5 minutes.
4. Serve hot.

Nutrition:

Calories 95; Total Fat 7.3 g; Saturated Fat 1 g

Cholesterol 0 mg; Sodium 148 mg; Total Carbs 7 g

Fiber 2.4 g; Sugar 1.6 g; Protein 2.7 g

61. Sautéed Kale

Preparation Time: 10 minutes

Cooking Time: 20 minutes

Servings: 4

Ingredients:

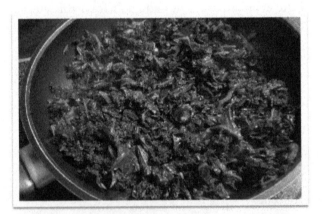

- 1 tablespoon extra-virgin olive oil
- 1 lemon, seeded and sliced thinly
- 1 onion, sliced thinly
- 3 garlic cloves, minced
- 2 pounds fresh kale, trimmed and chopped
- ½ cup scallions, chopped
- Sea salt and freshly ground black pepper, to taste

Directions:

1. In a large skillet, heat the oil over medium heat and cook the lemon slices for 5 minutes.
2. With a slotted spoon, remove the lemon slices from skillet and set aside.
3. In the same skillet, add the onion and garlic and sauté for about 5 minutes.
4. Add the kale, scallions, honey, salt, and pepper and cook for 8-10 minutes.
5. Add the lemon slices and mix until well combined.
6. Serve hot.

Nutrition:

Calories 161

Total Fat 3.6 g

Saturated Fat 0.5 g

Cholesterol 0 mg

Sodium 160 mg

Total Carbs 28.3 g

Fiber 4.6 g

Sugar 1.6 g

Protein 7.5 g

62.Parsley Mushrooms

Preparation Time: 15 minutes

Cooking Time: 14 minutes

Servings: 2

Ingredients:

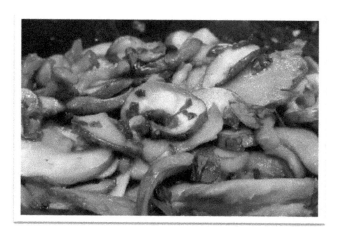

- 2 tablespoons olive oil
- 2-3 tablespoons onion, minced
- ½ teaspoon garlic, minced
- 12 ounces fresh mushrooms, sliced
- 1 tablespoon fresh parsley
- Sea salt and freshly ground black pepper, to taste

Directions:

1. In a skillet, heat the oil over medium heat and sauté the onion and garlic for 2-3 minutes.
2. Add the mushrooms and cook for 8-10 minutes or until desired doneness.
3. Stir in the parsley salt and black pepper and remove from the heat.
4. Serve hot.

Nutrition:

Calories 162

Total Fat 14.5 g

Saturated Fat 2 g

Cholesterol 0 mg

Sodium 128 mg

Total Carbs 6.9 g

Fiber 2 g

Sugar 3.4 g

Protein 5.6 g

63.Vegetarian Burgers

Preparation Time: 15 minutes

Cooking Time: 16 minutes

Servings: 4

Ingredients:

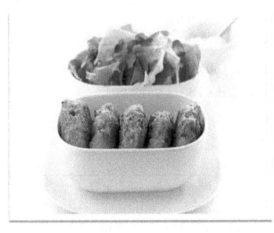

- 1-pound firm tofu, drained, pressed, and crumbled
- ¾ cup rolled oats
- ¼ cup flaxseeds
- 2 cups frozen spinach, thawed
- 1 medium onion, chopped finely
- 4 garlic cloves, minced
- 1 teaspoon ground cumin
- 1 teaspoon red pepper flakes, crushed
- Sea salt and freshly ground black pepper, to taste
- 2 tablespoons olive oil
- 6 cups fresh salad greens

Directions:

1. In a large bowl, add all the ingredients except oil and salad greens and mix until well combined.
2. Set aside for about 10 minutes.
3. Make desired size patties from mixture.
4. In a nonstick frying pan, heat the oil over medium heat and cook the patties for 6-8 minutes per side.
5. Serve these patties alongside the salad greens.

Nutrition:

Calories 185

Total Fat 10.2 g

Saturated Fat 1.7 g

Cholesterol 0 mg

Sodium 80 mg

Total Carbs 14.6 g

Fiber 5.1 g

Sugar 2.8 g

Protein 9.8 g

Dinner Recipes

64. Carrot and Golden Beet Soup

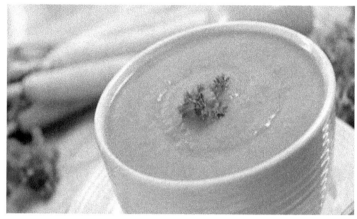

Nutrition:

Calories 248; Total Fat 15.7 g;

Saturated Fat 2.7 g; Cholesterol 75 mg;

Sodium 94 mg; Total Carbs 0.4 g

Fiber 0g; Sugar 0 g; Protein 24.9 g

Preparation Time: 5 minutes

Cooking Time: 30 minutes

Servings: 04

Ingredients:

- 6-7 carrots, chopped into 1/2-inch pieces
- 2-3 golden beets, chopped into 1/2-inch cubes
- 2 shallots, chopped into chunks
- 1 tablespoon olive oil
- 1/4 teaspoons ground turmeric, divided
- 1/4 teaspoons ground cumin, divided
- 1/2 teaspoons dried thyme, divided
- 1/2 teaspoons sea salt
- 2-3 cups vegetable stock
- 2-3 teaspoons lime juice

FOR SERVING:

- Chopped cilantro or parsley for serving, optional

Directions:

1. Layer 2 baking sheets with tin foil. Preheat the oven to 400 degrees F.
2. Add carrots, beet, and shallot to the baking sheets.
3. Top the veggies with spices, salt, and herbs.
4. Drizzle half tablespoon oil and cover the veggies with a foil sheet.
5. Bake for 30 minutes until al dente.
6. Transfer all the ingredients to a blender.
7. Puree the mixture and add the saucepan.

8. Cook for 1 minute.

9. Garnish with parsley.

10. Serve.

65. Sweet Potato Green Soup

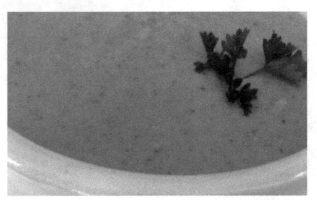

Preparation Time: 5 minutes

Cooking Time: 22 minutes

Servings: 2

Ingredients:

- 2 tablespoons coconut oil
- 1 large onion, chopped
- 3 cloves garlic, minced
- 2-in piece ginger, peeled and minced
- 3 cups bone broth
- 1 medium white sweet potato, cubed
- 1 large head broccoli, chopped
- 1 bunch kale, chopped
- 1 lemon, ½ zested and juice reserved
- ½ teaspoon sea salt
- 1 bunch cilantro

Directions:

1. Add and heat oil in a skillet. Stir in onions.

2. Sauté for 7 minutes then add ginger and garlic. Cook for 1 minute.

3. Stir in sweet potato, broccoli, and broth.

4. Boil the soup then reduce the heat to a simmer.

5. Cook for 15 minutes then turn off the heat.

6. Add all the remaining ingredients.

7. Puree the mixture using a handheld blender.

8. Garnish with cilantro.

9. Serve warm.

Nutrition:

Calories 249

Total Fat 11.9 g

Saturated Fat 1.7 g

Cholesterol 78 mg

Sodium 79 mg

Total Carbs 1.8 g

Fiber 1.1 g

Sugar 0.3 g

Protein 35 g

66. Lentil Spinach Soup

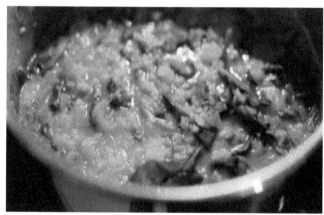

Nutrition:

Calories 301; Total Fat 12.2 g;

Saturated Fat 2.4 g; Cholesterol 110 mg;

Sodium 276 mg; Total Carbs 15 g;

Fiber 0.9 g; Sugar 1.4 g; Protein 28.8 g

Preparation Time: 05 minutes

Cooking Time: 15 minutes

Servings: 4

Ingredients:

- 1/2 onion
- 2 carrots
- 1 rib celery
- 1 clove garlic
- 1 cup tomatoes, diced
- 1 teaspoon dried vegetable broth powder
- 1 teaspoon Sazon seasoning
- 1 cup red lentils
- 1 tablespoon lemon juice
- 3 cups alkaline water
- 1 bunch spinach

Directions:

1. Add all the vegetables to a greased pan.
2. Sauté for 5 minutes then add broth, tomatoes, and Sazon seasoning.
3. Mix well and stir in red lentils along with water.

4. Cook until lentil is soft and tender.

5. Add spinach and cook for 2 minutes.

6. Serve warm with lemon slices on top.

67. Tangy Lentil Soup

Preparation Time: 5 minutes

Cooking Time: 15 minutes

Servings: 4

Ingredients:

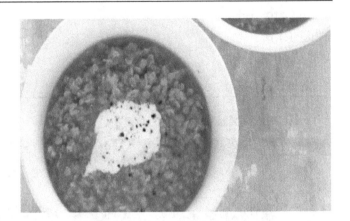

- 2 cups red lentils, picked over and rinsed
- 1 serrano Chile pepper, chopped
- 1 large tomato, roughly chopped
- 1 1 1/2-inch piece ginger, peeled and grated
- 3 cloves garlic, finely chopped
- 1/4 teaspoon ground turmeric
- Sea salt, to taste

TOPPING:

- 1/4 cup coconut yogurt

Directions:

1. Add lentils to a pot and with enough water to cover it.

2. Bring the lentils to a boil then reduce the heat.

3. Cook for 10 minutes on low simmer.

4. Stir in all the remaining ingredients.

5. Cook until lentils are soft and well mixed.

6. Garnish a dollop of coconut yogurt.

7. Serve.

Nutrition:

Calories 248; Total Fat 2.4 g; Saturated Fat 0.1 g

Cholesterol 320 mg; Sodium 350 mg; Total Carbs 12.2 g

Fiber 0.7 g; Sugar 0.7 g; Protein 44.3 g

68. Vegetable Casserole

Preparation Time: 5 minutes

Cooking Time: 1hr. 30 minutes

Servings: 06

Ingredients:

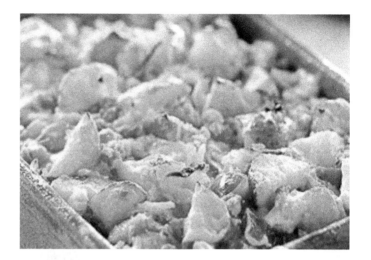

- 2 large eggplants, peeled and sliced
- Sea salt, to taste
- 2 large cucumbers, diced
- 2 small green peppers, diced
- 1 Small red pepper, diced
- 1 Small yellow pepper, diced
- ¼ lb. green beans, sliced
- ½ cup olive oil
- 2 large sweet onions, Chopped
- 3 cloves garlic, crushed
- 2 yellow Squash, cubed
- 20 cherry tomatoes, halved
- ½ teaspoon sea salt
- ¼ teaspoon fresh ground pepper
- ¼ lb. lima beans (Optional)
- A handful of fresh chopped basil (Optional)
- ¼ cup alkaline water
- 1 cup fresh seasoned breadcrumbs

Directions:

1. Set your oven to 350 degrees F. Mix eggplant with salt and keep it aside.
2. Heat a greased skillet and sauté eggplant until evenly browned.
3. Transfer the eggplant to a plate.
4. Sauté onions in the same pan until soft.
5. Stir in garlic and cook for a minute then turn off the heat.
6. Layer a greased casserole dish with eggplants, green beans, cucumbers, peppers and yellow squash.
7. Add tomatoes, onion mixture, salt, and pepper.
8. Sprinkle seasoned breadcrumbs on top.
9. Bake for 1 hour and 30 minutes.
10. Serve.

Nutrition:

Calories 372

Total Fat 11.1 g

Saturated Fat 5.8 g

Cholesterol 610 mg

Sodium 749 mg

Total Carbs 0.9 g

Fiber 0.2 g

Sugar 0.2 g

Protein 63.5 g

69. Mushroom Leek Soup

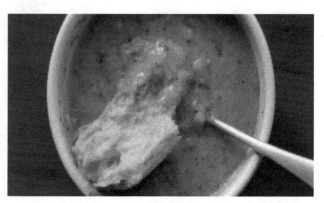

Preparation Time: 5 minutes

Cooking Time: 8 minutes

Servings: 4

Ingredients:

- 3 tablespoons vegetable oil, divided
- 2 ¾ cups leeks, finely chopped
- 3 garlic cloves, finely minced
- 7 cups assorted mushrooms, cleaned and sliced
- 5 tablespoons almond flour
- ¾ teaspoon sea salt
- ½ teaspoon ground black pepper
- 1 tablespoon fresh dill, very finely minced (optional)
- 3 cups vegetable broth
- 2/3 cup coconut cream
- ½ cup almond milk
- 1 ½ tablespoons sherry vinegar

Directions:

1. Heat oil in a Dutch oven and sauté garlic and leeks until soft.
2. Stir in mushrooms and sauté for 10 minutes.
3. Add flour, pepper, dill, and salt.
4. Mix well and cook for 2 minutes.
5. Pour in broth and cook to boil.
6. Reduce the heat and add the remaining ingredients.
7. Serve warm with almond flour bread.

Nutrition:

Calories 127; Total Fat 3.5 g; Saturated Fat 0.5 g

Cholesterol 162 mg; Sodium 142 mg; Total Carbs 3.6g

Fiber 0.4 g; Sugar 0.5 g; Protein 21.5 g

70. Red Lentil Squash Soup

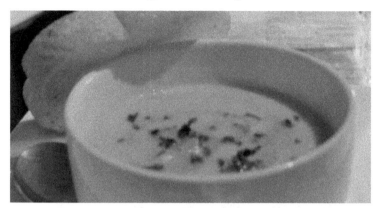

Preparation Time: 5 minutes

Cooking Time: 4 minutes

Servings: 04

Ingredients:

- 1 yellow onion, chopped
- 2 tablespoons olive oil
- 1 large butternut squash, diced
- 1 1/2 cups red lentils
- 2 teaspoons dried sage
- 7 cups vegetable broth
- mineral sea salt and white or fresh cracked pepper, to taste

Directions:

1. Heat oil in a large stockpot.
2. Add onions and cook for 5 minutes.
3. Stir in squash and sage. Cook for 3 to 5 minutes.
4. Add broth, salt, pepper, and lentils.
5. Cook for 30 minutes on low heat.
6. Puree the mixture using a handheld blender.
7. Garnish with parsley and serve.

Nutrition:

Calories 323; Total Fat 7.5 g; Saturated Fat 1.1 g

Cholesterol 20 mg; Sodium 97 mg; Total Carbs 21.4 g

Fiber 0 g; Sugar 0 g; Protein 10.1g

71. Cauliflower Potato Curry

Preparation Time: 10 minutes

Cooking Time: 35 minutes

Servings: 04

Ingredients:

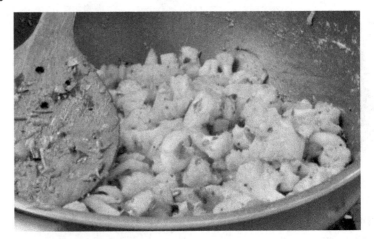

- 2 tablespoons vegetable oil
- 1 large onion, chopped
- a large piece of ginger, grated
- 3 garlic cloves, finely chopped
- ½ teaspoon turmeric
- 1 teaspoon ground cumin
- 1 teaspoon curry powder, or to taste
- 1 cup tomatoes, chopped
- ½ teaspoon sugar
- 1 cauliflower, cut into florets
- 2 potatoes, cut into chunks
- 1 small green chili, halved lengthways
- A squeeze of lemon juice
- Handful coriander, roughly chopped, to serve

Directions:

1. Add onion to a greased skillet and sauté until soft.
2. Stir in all the spices along with potatoes and cauliflower.
3. Sauté for 5 minutes then add tomatoes, sugar and green chilies.
4. Cover and cook for 30 minutes.
5. Serve warm with lemon juice and coriander.

Nutrition:

Calories 332

Total Fat 7.5 g

Saturated Fat 1.1 g

Cholesterol 20 mg

Sodium 97 mg

Total Carbs 19.4 g

Fiber 0 g

Sugar 0 g

Protein 3.1g

72. Vegetable Bean Curry

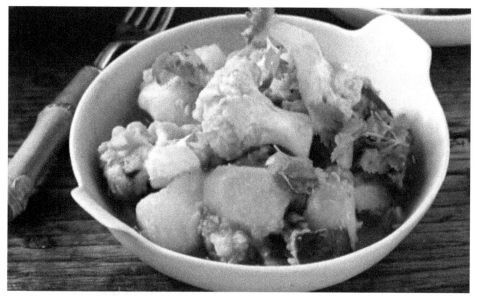

Preparation Time: 5 minutes

Cooking Time: 6 hours

Servings: 08

Ingredients:

- 1 onion, finely chopped
- 4 garlic cloves, chopped
- 3 teaspoons coriander powder
- 1-1/2 teaspoons cinnamon powder
- 1 teaspoon ginger powder
- 1 teaspoon turmeric powder
- 1/2 teaspoon cayenne pepper
- 2 tablespoons tomato paste
- 1 tablespoon avocado oil
- 2 cans (15 ounces each) lima beans, rinsed and drained

- 3 cups sweet potatoes, cubed peeled
- 3 cups fresh cauliflower florets
- 4 medium carrots, diced
- 2 medium tomatoes, seeded and chopped
- 2 cups vegetable broth
- 1 cup light coconut milk
- 1/2 teaspoon pepper
- 1/4 teaspoon sea salt

Directions:

1. Heat oil in a slow cooker and add all the vegetables.
2. Stir in all the remaining ingredients.
3. Cook for 5 to 6 hours on low-temperature settings.
4. Serve warm.

Nutrition:

Calories 403; Total Fat 12.5 g; Saturated Fat 1.1 g

Cholesterol 20 mg; Sodium 397 mg; Total Carbs 21.4 g

Fiber 0 g; Sugar 0 g; Protein 8.1g

73. Wild mushroom soup

Preparation Time: 10 minutes

Cooking Time: 15 minutes

Servings: 04

Ingredients:

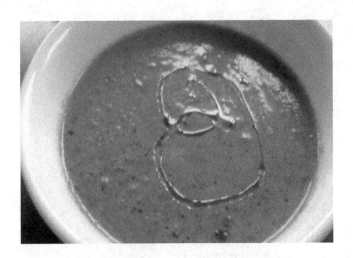

- 4 oz. almond butter
- 1 shallot, chopped
- 5 oz. portabella mushrooms, chopped
- 5 oz. oyster mushrooms, chopped
- 5 oz. shiitake mushrooms, chopped
- 1 garlic clove, minced
- ½ teaspoon dried thyme
- 3 cups alkaline water
- 1 vegetable bouillon cube
- 1 cup coconut cream
- ½ lb. celery root, chopped

- 1 tablespoon white wine vinegar
- Fresh parsley (optional)

Directions:

1. Melt butter in a cooking pan over medium heat.
2. Add vegetables to the pan and sauté until golden brown.
3. Stir in all the remaining ingredients to the pan and boil the mixture.
4. Reduce the heat to low and let it simmer for 15 minutes.
5. Add cream to the soup and puree it, using a hand-held blender.
6. Serve warm with chopped parsley on top.

Nutrition:

Calories 243

Total Fat 7.5 g

Saturated Fat 1.1 g

Cholesterol 20 mg

Sodium 357 mg

Total Carbs 14.4 g

Fiber 0 g

Sugar 0 g

Protein 10.1g

74. Quinoa, Bean, and Mango Salad

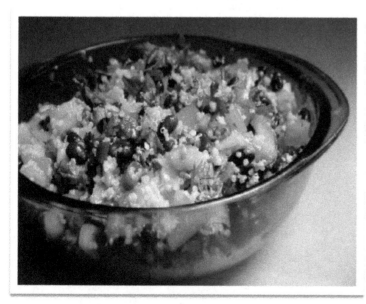

Nutrition:

Calories 367; Total Fat 8.7 g;

Saturated Fat 1.2 g; Cholesterol 0 mg;

Sodium 375 mg; Total Carbs 61 g

Fiber 12.7 g; Sugar 11.3 g; Protein 15.1 g

Preparation Time: 15 minutes

Cooking Time: 0 minutes

Servings: 4

Ingredients:

- 2 cups cooked black beans
- 1 cup cooked quinoa
- 1½ cups fresh mango, peeled, pitted, and chopped

- 1 large red bell pepper, seeded and chopped
- ½ cup fresh cilantro, chopped
- ¼ cup scallion, chopped
- 1 small jalapeño pepper, seeded and chopped finely
- 2 garlic cloves, minced
- 2 tablespoons fresh lemon juice
- 1½ tablespoons olive oil
- Sea salt, to taste

Directions:

1. In a large bowl, add all the ingredients and gently stir to combine.
2. Refrigerate for about 1-2 hours before serving.

Nutrition:

Calories 367; Total Fat 8.7 g; Saturated Fat 1.2 g

Cholesterol 0 mg; Sodium 375 mg; Total Carbs 61 g

Fiber 12.7 g; Sugar 11.3 g; Protein 15.1 g

75. Mixed Bean Salad

Preparation Time: 15 minutes

Cooking Time: 0 minutes

Servings: 8

Ingredients:

FOR SALAD:

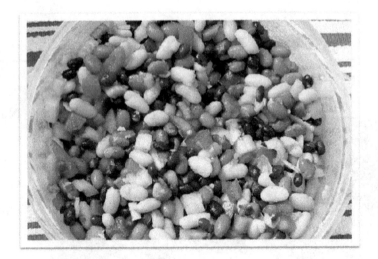

- 1½ cups cooked cannellini beans
- 1½ cups cooked red kidney beans
- 1½ cups cooked black beans
- 2 cups cucumber, chopped
- 1 cup onion, chopped
- 1½ cups plum tomato, chopped

FOR DRESSING:

- 1 garlic clove, minced
- 2 tablespoons shallots, minced
- 2 teaspoons lemon zest, grated finely
- ¼ cup fresh lime juice
- 2 tablespoons extra-virgin olive oil

- Sea salt and freshly ground black pepper, to taste

Directions:

1. For salad: in a large serving bowl, add the couscous and remaining ingredients and stir to combine.
2. For dressing: in another small bowl, add all the ingredients and beat until well combined.
3. Pour the dressing over the salad and gently toss to coat well.
4. Serve immediately.

Nutrition:

Calories 327

Total Fat 4.5 g

Saturated Fat 0.7 g

Cholesterol 0 mg

Sodium 46 mg

Total Carbs 54.9 g

Fiber 15.4 g

Sugar 3.5 g

Protein 19.4 g

76. Quinoa and Lentil Soup

Preparation Time: 15 minutes

Cooking Time: 30 minutes

Servings: 6

Ingredients:

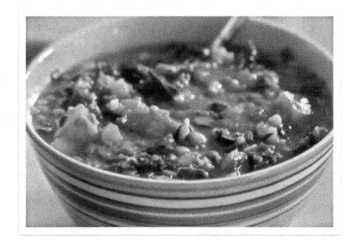

- 1 tablespoon coconut oil
- 3 carrots, peeled and chopped
- 3 celery stalks, chopped
- 1 yellow onion, chopped
- 4 garlic cloves, minced
- 4 cups tomatoes, chopped
- 1 cup red lentils, rinsed and drained
- ½ cup dried quinoa, rinsed and drained
- 1½ teaspoons ground cumin
- 1 teaspoon red chili powder
- 6 cups homemade vegetable broth
- 2 cups fresh spinach, chopped

Directions:

1. In a large pan, heat the oil over medium heat and sauté the celery, onion, and carrot for 4-5 minutes.
2. Add the garlic and sauté for about 1 minute.
3. Add the remaining ingredients except spinach and bring to a boil.
4. Reduce the heat to low and simmer, covered for 20 minutes.
5. Stir in spinach and simmer for 3-4 minutes.
6. Serve hot.

Nutrition:

Calories 275

Total Fat 5.4 g

Saturated Fat 2.6 g

Cholesterol 0 mg

Sodium 714 mg

Total Carbs 40.4 g

Fiber 13.9 g

Sugar 7 g

Protein 17.2 g

77. Lentil and Veggie Soup

Preparation Time: 15 minutes

Cooking Time: 1 hour 15 minutes

Servings: 8

Ingredients:

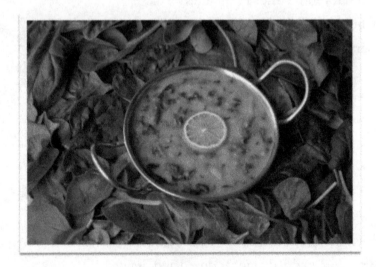

- 2 tablespoons olive oil
- 2 carrots, peeled and chopped
- 2 celery stalks, chopped
- 2 sweet onions, chopped
- 3 garlic cloves, minced
- 1¾ cups brown lentils, rinsed
- 2½ cups tomatoes, finely chopped
- ¼ teaspoon dried basil, crushed
- ¼ teaspoon dried oregano, crushed
- ¼ teaspoon dried thyme, crushed

- 1 teaspoon ground cumin
- ½ teaspoon ground coriander
- ½ teaspoon paprika
- 6 cups homemade vegetable broth
- 3 cups fresh spinach, chopped
- Sea salt and freshly ground black pepper, to taste
- 2 tablespoons fresh lemon juice

Directions:

1. In a large soup pan, heat the oil over medium heat and sauté carrot, celery, and onion for 5 minutes.
2. Add the garlic, sauté for about 1 minute.
3. Add the lentils and sauté for 3 minutes.
4. Stir in the tomatoes, herbs, spices, and broth and bring to a boil.
5. Reduce the heat to low and simmer, partially covered for about 1 hour or until desired doneness
6. Stir in the spinach, salt and black pepper and cook for 4 minutes.
7. Stir in the lemon juice and serve hot.

Nutrition:

Calories 275; Total Fat 6.1 g; Saturated Fat 0.9 g

Cholesterol 0 mg; Sodium 645 mg; Total Carbs 39.7 g

Fiber 10.4 g; Sugar 9.8 g; Protein 18.1 g

78. Mixed Mushroom Stew

Preparation Time: 15 minutes

Cooking Time: 15 minutes

Servings: 4

Ingredients:

- 2 tablespoons olive oil
- 2 onions, chopped
- 3 garlic cloves, minced
- ½ pound fresh button mushrooms, chopped
- ¼ pound fresh shiitake mushrooms, chopped

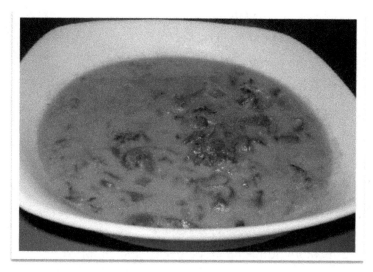

- ¼ pound fresh Portobello mushrooms, chopped
- Sea salt and freshly ground black pepper, to taste
- ¼ cup homemade vegetable broth
- ½ cup coconut milk
- 2 tablespoons fresh parsley, chopped

Directions:

1. In a large skillet, heat oil over medium heat and sauté the onion and garlic for 4-5 minutes.
2. Add the mushrooms, salt, and black pepper and cook for 4-5 minutes.
3. Add the broth and coconut milk and bring to a gentle boil.
4. Simmer for 4-5 minutes or until desired doneness.
5. Stir in the cilantro and remove from heat.
6. Serve hot.

Nutrition:

Calories 182; Total Fat 14.7 g; Saturated Fat 7.4 g;

Cholesterol 0 mg; Sodium 90 mg; Total Carbs 11.5 g

Fiber 3.1 g; Sugar 5.4 g; Protein 5.4 g

79. Veggie Stew

Preparation Time: 20 minutes

Cooking Time: 35 minutes

Servings: 8

Ingredients:

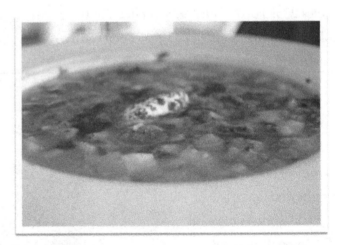

- 2 tablespoons coconut oil
- 1 large sweet onion, chopped
- 1 medium parsnip, peeled and chopped
- 3 tablespoons tomato paste
- 2 large garlic cloves, minced
- ½ teaspoon ground cinnamon
- ½ teaspoon ground ginger
- 1 teaspoon ground cumin
- ¼ teaspoon cayenne pepper
- 2 medium carrots, peeled and chopped
- 2 medium purple potatoes, peeled and chopped
- 2 medium sweet potatoes, peeled and chopped

- 4 cups vegetable broth
- 2 tablespoons fresh lemon juice
- 2 cups fresh kale, trimmed and chopped
- ¼ cup fresh cilantro leaves, chopped
- 3 tablespoons coconut cream

Directions:

1. In a large soup pan, melt the coconut oil over medium-high heat and sauté the onion for about 5 minutes.
2. Add the parsnip and sauté for 3 minutes.
3. Stir in the tomato paste, garlic, and spices and sauté for 2 minutes.
4. Stir in carrots, potatoes, sweet potatoes, and broth and bring to a boil.
5. Reduce the heat to medium-low and simmer, covered for about 20 minutes.
6. Stir in the lemon juice and kale and simmer for 5 minutes.
7. Serve with a topping of coconut cream and cilantro.

Nutrition:

Calories 225; Total Fat 6.7 g; Saturated Fat 5.9 g

Cholesterol 0 mg; Sodium 306 mg; Total Carbs 39.5 g

Fiber 5.5 g; Sugar 14.4 g; Protein 3.1 g

80. Bean and Veggie Chili

Preparation Time: 20 minutes

Cooking Time: 2 hours 10 minutes

Servings: 5

Ingredients:

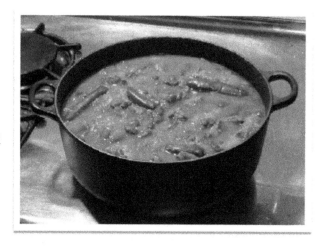

- 2 tablespoons olive oil
- 1 onion, chopped
- 1 large green bell pepper, seeded and sliced
- 4 garlic cloves, minced
- 2 jalapeño peppers, sliced
- 1 teaspoon ground cumin
- 1 teaspoon cayenne pepper
- 1 tablespoon red chili powder
- 2 cups tomatoes, finely chopped
- 4 cups cooked black beans

- 2 cups homemade vegetable broth
- Sea salt and freshly ground black pepper, to taste

Directions:

1. In a large pan, heat the oil over medium-high heat and sauté the onion and bell peppers for 3-4 minutes.
2. Add the garlic, jalapeño peppers, and spices and sauté for about 1 minute.
3. Add the sweet potato and cook for 4-5 minutes.
4. Add the remaining ingredients except the pita chips and bring to a boil.
5. Reduce the heat to medium-low and simmer, covered for about 1½-2 hours.
6. Season with the salt and black pepper and serve hot with a topping of pita chips.

Nutrition:

Calories 285; Total Fat 7.7 g; Saturated Fat 1 g

Cholesterol 0 mg; Sodium 700 mg; Total Carbs 43 g

Fiber 15.4 g; Sugar 6.3 g; Protein 16.4 g

81. Lentil Chili

Preparation Time: 15 minutes

Cooking Time: 2 hours 40 minutes

Servings: 8

Ingredients:

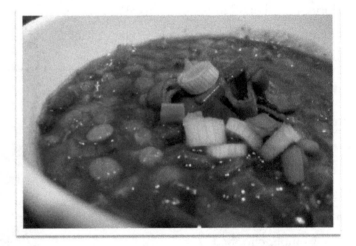

- 2 teaspoons olive oil
- 1 large onion, chopped
- 3 medium carrots, peeled and chopped
- 4 celery stalks, chopped
- 2 garlic cloves, minced
- 1 jalapeño pepper, seeded and chopped
- ½ tablespoon dried thyme, crushed
- 1 tablespoon chipotle chili powder
- ½ tablespoon cayenne pepper
- 1½ tablespoons ground coriander
- 1½ tablespoons ground cumin
- 1 teaspoon ground turmeric
- Sea salt and freshly ground black pepper, to taste
- 1-pound red lentils, rinsed

- 8 cups homemade vegetable broth
- ½ cup scallion, chopped

Directions:

1. In a large pan, heat the oil over medium heat and sauté the onion, carrot, and celery for 5 minutes.
2. Add the garlic, jalapeño pepper, thyme, and spices and sauté for about 1 minute.
3. Add the tomato paste, lentils, and broth and bring to a boil.
4. Reduce the heat to low and simmer for 2-2½ hours.
5. Serve hot with a garnish of scallion.

Nutrition:

Calories 280

Total Fat 3.7 g

Saturated Fat 0.7 g

Cholesterol 0 mg

Sodium 822 mg

Total Carbs 41.5 g

Fiber 19.3 g

Sugar 4.3 g

Protein 20.5 g

82. Kidney Bean Curry

Preparation Time: 15 minutes

Cooking Time: 25 minutes

Servings: 6

Ingredients:

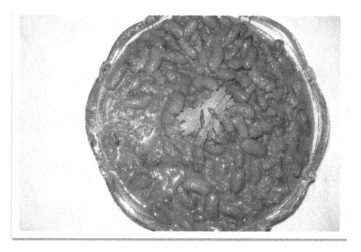

- 4 tablespoons olive oil
- 1 medium onion, chopped finely
- 2 garlic cloves, minced
- 2 tablespoons fresh ginger, minced
- 1 teaspoon ground coriander
- 1 teaspoon ground cumin
- ½ teaspoon ground turmeric
- ¼ teaspoon cayenne pepper
- Sea salt and freshly ground black pepper, to taste
- 2 large plum tomatoes, chopped finely

- 3 cups cooked red kidney beans
- 2 cups water
- ¼ cup fresh cilantro, chopped

Directions:

1. In a large pan, heat the oil over medium heat and sauté the onion, garlic, and ginger for 6-8 minutes.
2. Stir in the spices cook for about 1-2 minutes.
3. Stir in the tomatoes, kidney beans, and water and bring to a boil over high heat.
4. Reduce the heat to medium and simmer for 10-15 minutes or until desired thickness.
5. Serve hot with a garnish of parsley.

Nutrition:

Calories 213; Total Fat 10.2 g; Saturated Fat 1.4 g

Cholesterol 0 mg; Sodium 222 mg; Total Carbs 24 g

Fiber 7 g; Sugar 3 g; Protein 8.5 g

83. Pumpkin Curry

Preparation Time: 15 minutes

Cooking Time: 35 minutes

Servings: 4

Ingredients:

FOR ROASTED PUMPKIN:

- 1 medium sugar pumpkin, peeled and cubed
- Sea salt, to taste
- 1 teaspoon olive oil

FOR CURRY:

- 1 teaspoon olive oil
- 1 onion, chopped
- 1 tablespoon fresh ginger, minced
- 1 tablespoon garlic, minced
- 1 cup coconut milk
- 2 cups vegetable broth
- 1 tablespoon curry powder
- 1 teaspoon ground cumin
- ½ teaspoon ground turmeric

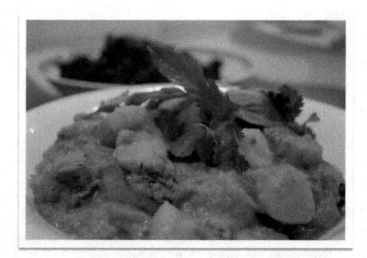

- Sea salt and freshly ground black pepper, to taste
- 1 tablespoon fresh lime juice
- 2 tablespoons fresh parsley, chopped

Directions:

1. Preheat the oven to 400 degrees F. Line a large baking sheet with parchment paper.
2. In a large bowl, add all ingredients for the roasted pumpkin and toss to coat well.
3. Place pumpkin onto prepared baking sheet in a single layer.
4. Roast for 20-25 minutes, flipping once halfway through.
5. Meanwhile, in a large pan, heat oil for the curry on medium-high heat.
6. Add onion and sauté for 4-5 minutes.
7. Add ginger and garlic and sauté for about 1 minute.
8. Add coconut milk, broth, spices, salt, and black pepper and bring to a boil.
9. Reduce the heat to low and simmer for 10 minutes.
10. Stir in the roasted pumpkin and simmer for 10 more minutes.
11. Serve hot with a garnish of parsley.

Nutrition:

Calories 263; Total Fat 18.3 g; Saturated Fat 13.5 g

Cholesterol 0 mg; Sodium 462 mg; Total Carbs 23.3 g

Fiber 7.8 g; Sugar 9.3 g; Protein 6.6 g

84. Tofu with Broccoli

Nutrition:

Calories 184; Total Fat 14.1 g;
Saturated Fat 8.9 g; Cholesterol 0 mg;
Sodium 35 mg; Total Carbs 63.6 g
Fiber 7.1 g; Sugar 1.8 g; Protein 11.2 g

Preparation Time: 15 minutes

Cooking Time: 13 minutes

Servings: 3

Ingredients:

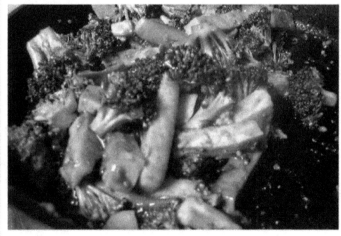

- 1 (12-ounce) package firm tofu, drained, pressed, and cut into 5 slices
- 2 tablespoons coconut oil, divided
- 2 cups small broccoli florets

- ¼ cup water
- ½ tablespoon garlic, minced
- ½ tablespoon fresh ginger, minced
- Freshly ground black pepper, to taste

Directions:

1. In a large non-stick skillet, melt 1 tablespoon of the coconut oil over medium-high heat and cook the tofu for 4-5 minutes per side or until crispy.
2. With a slotted spoon, scoop the tofu slices onto a paper towel-lined plate to absorb any extra oil.
3. Then, cut each tofu slice into equal sized pieces.
4. Meanwhile, in a large microwave-safe bowl, add the broccoli florets and water.
5. Cover the bowl and microwave on high for about 5 minutes.
6. Remove from the microwave and drain the broccoli.
7. In the same skillet, melt the remaining coconut oil over medium heat and sauté the garlic and ginger for about 1 minute.
8. Add the tofu, broccoli and black pepper and cook for 2 minutes, tossing occasionally.
9. Remove from the heat and serve hot.

85. Black-Eyed Pea Curry

Preparation Time: 15 minutes

Cooking Time: 15 minutes

Servings: 3

Ingredients:

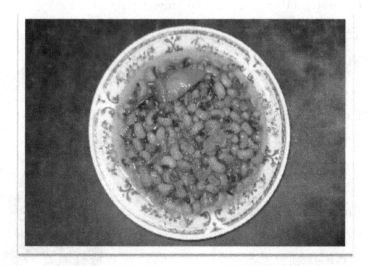

- 1 teaspoon olive oil
- 1 onion, chopped
- 2 teaspoons fresh ginger, minced
- 3 garlic cloves, minced
- 2 green chilies, split in half
- 1 tablespoon fresh thyme, chopped
- 2 teaspoons curry powder
- ½ teaspoon ground cumin
- 1 (16-ounce) can black-eyed peas, drained and rinsed
- ¾ cup water
- ¾ cup coconut milk
- 1 teaspoon applesauce

- 1 tablespoon fresh lime juice
- Sea salt and freshly ground black pepper, to taste
- 2 tablespoons fresh parsley, chopped

Directions:

1. In a pan, heat the oil over medium heat and sauté the onion for 4-5 minutes.
2. Add the ginger, garlic, green chili, thyme, curry powder, and cumin and sauté for about 1 minute.
3. Add the black-eyed peas, water, coconut milk, and applesauce and bring to a boil.
4. Cover and cook for 5 minutes.
5. Stir in the lime juice, salt, and black pepper and cook or about 1 minute.
6. Remove from the heat and serve hot with a garnish of parsley.

Nutrition:

Calories 297; Total Fat 17.6 g; Saturated Fat 13 g

Cholesterol 0 mg; Sodium 126 mg; Total Carbs 30.4 g

Fiber 8.2 g; Sugar 3.9 g; Protein 9.9 g

86. Chickpea Mashed Potatoes

Preparation Time: 5 minutes

Cooking Time: 30 minutes

Servings: 4

Ingredients:

- 2 cups chickpeas, cooked
- ¼ cup green onions, diced
- 2 teaspoons sea salt
- 2 teaspoons onion powder
- 1 cup walnut milk; homemade, unsweetened

Directions:

1. Plug in a food processor, add chickpeas to it, pour in the milk, and then add salt and onion powder.
2. Cover the blending jar with its lid and then pulse for 1 to 2 minutes until smooth; blend in water if the mixture is too thick.
3. Take a medium saucepan, place it over medium heat, and then add a blended chickpea mixture.
4. Stir green onions into the chickpeas mixture and then cook the mixture for 30 minutes, stirring constantly.
5. Serve straight away.

Nutrition: Calories: 145.8

Carbohydrates: 19.1 grams

Fat: 7.3 grams

Protein: 3.3 grams

87. Mushroom and Onion Gravy

Preparation Time: 5 minutes

Cooking Time: 18 minutes

Servings: 4

Ingredients:

- 1 cup sliced onions, chopped
- 1 cup mushrooms, sliced
- 2 teaspoons onion powder
- 2 teaspoons sea salt
- 1 teaspoon dried thyme
- 6 tablespoons chickpea flour
- ½ teaspoon cayenne pepper
- 1 teaspoon dried oregano
- 4 tablespoons grapeseed oil
- 4 cups spring water

Directions:

1. Take a medium pot, place it over medium-high heat, add oil and when hot, add onions and mushrooms, and then cook for 1 minute.
2. Season the vegetables with onion powder, salt, thyme, and oregano. Stir until mixed, and cook for 5 minutes.
3. Pour in water, stir in cayenne pepper, stir well, and then bring the mixture to a boil.
4. Slowly stir in chickpea flour, and bring the mixture to a boil again.
5. Remove pan from heat and then serve gravy with a favorite dish.

Nutrition:

Calories: 120

Carbohydrates: 8.4 grams

Fat: 7.6 grams

Protein: 2.2 grams

88. Vegetable Chili

Preparation Time: 5 minutes

Cooking Time: 30 minutes

Servings: 6

Ingredients:

- 2 cups black beans, cooked
- 1 medium red bell pepper; deseeded, chopped
- 1 poblano chili; deseeded, chopped
- 2 jalapeño chilies; deseeded, chopped
- 4 tablespoons cilantro, chopped
- 1 large white onion; peeled, chopped
- 1 ½ tablespoon minced garlic
- 1 ½ teaspoon sea salt
- 1 ½ teaspoon cumin powder
- 1 ½ teaspoon red chili powder
- 3 teaspoons lime juice
- 2 tablespoons grapeseed oil
- 2 ½ cups vegetable stock

Directions:

1. Take a large pot, place it over medium-high heat, add oil and when hot, add onion and cook for 4–5 minutes until translucent.
2. Add bell pepper, jalapeno pepper, poblano chili, and garlic and then cook for 3–4 minutes until veggies turn tender.
3. Season the vegetables with salt, stir in cumin powder and red chili powder, and then add chickpeas and vegetable stock.
4. Bring the mixture to a boil, then switch heat to medium-low and simmer the chili for 15–20 minutes until thickened slightly.
5. Then remove the pot from heat, spoon chili stew among six bowls, drizzle with lime juice, garnish with cilantro, and serve.

Nutrition: Calories: 224.2

Carbs: 42.6 grams

Fat: 1.2 grams

Protein: 12.5 grams

89. Spinach with Chickpeas and Lemon

Preparation Time: 5 minutes

Cooking Time: 10 minutes

Servings: 2

Ingredients:

- 3 tbsp oil
- 1 onion, thinly slices
- 4 garlic cloves, minced
- 1 tbsp ginger, grated
- 1/2 container cherry tomatoes
- 1 lemon, freshly zested and juiced
- 1 tbsp red pepper flakes, crushed
- 1 can chickpeas
- Salt to taste

Directions:

1. Add oil in a skillet and cook onions until browned. Add garlic cloves, ginger, tomatoes, zest, and pepper flakes. Cook for 4 minutes.
2. Add chickpeas and cook for 3 more minutes. Add spinach and cook until they start to wilt.
3. Add lemon juice and season with salt to taste. Cook for 2 more minutes.
4. Serve and enjoy.

Nutrition:

Calories: 209

Total fat: 8.1 grams

Saturated fat: 1 grams

Total carbohydrates: 28.5 grams

Protein: 22.5 grams

Fiber: 6 grams

Sodium: 372 milligrams

Potassium: 286 milligrams

90. Raw Green Veggie Soup

Preparation Time: 5 minutes

Cooking Time: 5 minutes

Servings: 1

Ingredients:

- 1 avocado
- 1 zucchini, chopped
- 2 celery stalks, chopped
- 2 cups spinach
- 1/4 cup parsley, fresh
- 2 slices green pepper
- 1/8 onion, chopped
- 1 garlic clove
- 1/4 cup almonds, soak overnight and rinse
- Salt to taste
- 1-1/2 cup water
- 1 lemon juice
- Diced watermelon radish for garnish

Directions:

1. Add all the ingredients in a food processor except salt.
2. Pulse until smooth or until the desired consistency is desired.
3. Pour the soup in a sauce pan to warm a little bit before seasoning with salt and squeezing lemon.
4. Garnish with watermelon radish and enjoy.

Nutrition:

Calories 48.9

Total fat 0.4 grams

Saturated fat 0.1 grams

Total carbs 10.6grams

Net carbs 6.7grams

Protein 3.1grams

Sugars 1.9grams

Fiber 3.9grams

Sodium 619 milligrams

Potassium 417 milligrams

91. Kale Caesar Salad

Preparation Time: 5 minutes

Cooking Time: 12 minutes

Servings: 1

Ingredients:

- 1 bunch of curly kale, washed
- 1 cup sunflower seeds
- 1/3 cup almond nuts
- 1/8 tbsp chipotle powder
- 2 garlic cloves
- 1-1/4 water
- 1-1/2 tbsp agave syrup
- 1/2 tbsp sea salt

Directions:

1. Wash and pat dry the curly kale; remove the center membrane. Tear the kale leaves into small sizes.
2. Add all other ingredients in a blender and blend until smooth and creamy.
3. Pour half of the mixture over the kale and toss until well coated.
4. Pour the remaining mixture and mix until the kales are well coated on the curls and folds.
5. Let rest for 10 minutes then serve on plates. Sprinkle sunflower seeds and enjoy.

Nutrition:

Calories: 157

Total fat: 6 gr

Saturated fat: 2 gr

Total carbohydrates: 18 gr

Protein: 9 gr

Sugar: 1 gr

Fiber: 2 gr

Sodium: 356 mg

92. Red and White Salad

Preparation Time: 5 minutes

Cooking Time: 10 minutes

Servings: 2

Ingredients:

- 3 radishes
- 1 fennel bulb, greens removed

- 1/2 jicama, peeled and halved
- 2 celery stalks
- Juice from 1 lime
- 1/4 cup avocado oil
- Salt to taste
- Macadamia nuts

Directions:

1. Slice radish, fennel, jicama and celery using a mandolin slicer on the thinnest setting.
2. Toss them in a mixing bowl with lime and oil. Season with salt then top with nuts.
3. Enjoy.

Nutrition:

Calories: 197

Total fat: 9 grams

Saturated fat: 4 grams

Total carbs: 20 grams

Protein: 7 grams

Sugars: 1 gram

Fiber: 2 grams

Sodium: 366 milligrams

93. Almond Milk

Preparation Time: 5 minutes

Cooking Time: 10 minutes

Servings: 2

Ingredients:

1. 1.7oz almonds, sliced
2. 133.8 oz filtered water
3. 1 tbsp sunflower granules
4. 2 dates, stones removed

Directions:

1. Soak the almonds for a few hours ahead of time.
2. Add all the ingredients in a blender and blend for 2 minutes.
3. Pour the milk in a container through a straining cloth. Carry in your lunch box or store in a fridge for up to 3 days.

4. You can use almond pulp in cakes or almond mixes.

Nutrition:

Calories 90

Total fat: 2.5 gr

Total carbohydrates: 16 gr

Protein: 1 gr

Sugars: 4 gr

Sodium: 140 mg

Potassium: 140 mg

94. Creamy Kale Salad with Avocado And Tomato

Preparation Time: 5 minutes

Cooking Time: 10 minutes

Servings: 2

Ingredients:

- 2 handful of kale
- 2 cherry tomatoes
- 1 ripe avocado
- Juice from 1 lime
- 1 garlic clove, crushed
- 1 tbsp agave
- 1/2 tbsp paprika
- 1/2 tbsp black pepper

Directions:

1. Wash kale and tomatoes and roughly chop them. Place them in a mixing bowl.
2. Peel the avocado and add it to the mixing bowl.
3. Add lemon juice and the rest of the ingredients to the bowl and mix them thoroughly.
4. Serve and enjoy.

Nutrition:

Calories: 179.2

Total fat: 14.1 grams

Saturated fat: 1.9grams

Total carbohydrates: 13.5grams

Protein: 3.7grams

Sugars: 6grams

Fiber: 6.1grams

Sodium: 77 milligrams

Potassium: 624 milligrams

95. Creamy Broccoli Soup

Preparation Time: 5 minutes

Cooking Time: 10 minutes

Servings: 5

Ingredients:

- 2 cups vegetable stock
- 4 cups broccoli, chopped
- 1 red pepper, chopped
- 1 avocado
- 2 onions, chopped
- 2 celery stalks, sliced
- Ginger to taste
- 1 tbsp salt

Directions:

1. Warm vegetable stock in a small pot. Add broccoli and season with salt to taste. Simmer for 5 minutes.
2. Add the broccoli in a blender with pepper, avocado, onions, and celery stalks. Add some water for thinning then blend until smooth.
3. Serve when warm with ginger to your liking. Garnish with a lemon slice. Enjoy.

Nutrition:

Calories: 270

Total fat: 18 grams

Saturated fat: 11 grams

Total carbohydrates: 17 grams

Protein: 12 grams

Sugars: 5 grams

Fiber: 3.5 grams

Sodium: 470 milligrams

96. Capress Stuffed Avocado

Preparation Time: 5 minutes

Cooking Time: 10 minutes

Servings: 4

Ingredients:

- 1/2 cup cherry tomatoes
- 4 0z baby bocconcini balls
- 2 tbsp basil pesto
- 1 tbsp minced garlic
- 1/4 oil
- Salt and pepper to taste
- 2 ripe avocados
- 2 tbsp balsamic glaze
- Basil for serving

Directions:

1. In a mixing bowl, add cherry tomatoes, bocconcini balls, basil pesto, garlic, salt and pepper to taste. Toss until well combined and all flavors have blended.
2. Half the avocados and arrange them on a platter.
3. Spoon the mixture in the avocado halves and drizzle with balsamic glaze.
4. Top with basil and serve. Enjoy.

Nutrition:

Calories: 341

Total fat: 29grams

Saturated fat: 7grams

Total carbohydrates: 15grams

Protein: 8 grams

Sugars: 4 grams

Fiber: 6 grams

Sodium: 220 milligrams

Potassium: 550 milligrams

Dessert Recipes

97. Baked Apples

Preparation Time: 15 minutes

Cooking Time: 18 minutes.

Servings: 4

Ingredients:

- 4 apples, cored
- ¼ cup coconut oil, softened
- 4 tsp ground cinnamon
- 1/8 tsp ground ginger
- 1/8 tsp ground nutmeg

Directions:

1. Preheat the oven to 350 degrees F.
2. Fill each apple with 1 tablespoon of coconut oil.
3. Sprinkle each with spices evenly.
4. Arrange the apples on a baking sheet.
5. Bake for about 12-18 minutes.

Nutrition: Calories 240; Total Fat 14.1 g; Saturated Fat 11.8 g; Cholesterol 0 mg; Sodium 2 mg; Total Carbs 32.7 g; Fiber 6.6 g; Sugar 23.3 g; Protein 0.7 g

Berries Granita

Preparation Time: 15 minutes

Cooking Time: 0 minutes

Servings: 4

Ingredients:

- ½ cup fresh strawberries, hulled and sliced
- ½ cup fresh raspberries
- ½ cup fresh blueberries
- ½ cup fresh blackberries
- 1 tbsp pure maple syrup
- 1 tbsp fresh lemon juice
- 1 cup ice cubes, crushed
- 1 tsp fresh mint leaves

Directions:

1. In a high-speed blender, add the berries, maple syrup, lemon juice, and ice cubes and pulse on high speed until smooth.
2. Transfer the berries mixture into an 8x8-inch baking dish evenly and freeze for at least 30 minutes.
3. Remove from the freezer and stir the granita completely using a fork.
4. Return it to the freezer and freeze it for about 2-3 hours. Scrape it every 30 minutes with a fork.
5. Place the granita into serving glasses and serve immediately garnished with mint leaves.

Nutrition: Calories 46; Total Fat 0.3 g; Saturated Fat 0 g; Cholesterol 0 mg; Sodium 4 mg; Total Carbs 11.1 g; Fiber 2.8 g; Sugar 7.3 g; Protein 0.7 g

98. Pumpkin Ice Cream

Preparation Time: 15 minutes.

Cooking Time: 0 minutes   Note: This recipe calls for the use of an ice cream machine

Servings: 6

Ingredients:

- 15 oz homemade pumpkin puree
- ½ cup dates, pitted and chopped
- 2 (14-oz) cans unsweetened coconut milk
- ½ tsp organic vanilla extract
- 1½ tsp pumpkin pie spice
- ½ tsp ground cinnamon
- Pinch of sea salt

Directions:

1. In a high-speed blender, add all the ingredients and pulse until smooth.
2. Transfer into an airtight container and freeze for about 1-2 hours.
3. Now, transfer the mixture into an ice cream maker and process it according to the manufacturer's directions.
4. Return the ice cream to the airtight container and freeze for about 1-2 hours before serving.

Nutrition: Calories 293; Total Fat 22.5 g; Saturated Fat 20.1 g; Cholesterol 0 mg; Sodium 99 mg; Total Carbs 24.8 g; Fiber 3.6 g; Sugar 14.1 g; Protein 2.3 g

99. Lemon Sorbet

Preparation Time: 10 minutes.

Cooking Time: 0 minutes

Servings: 4

Note: This recipe calls for the use of an ice cream maker

Ingredients:

- 2 tbsp fresh lemon zest, grated
- ½ cup pure maple syrup
- 2 cups water
- 1½ cups fresh lemon juice

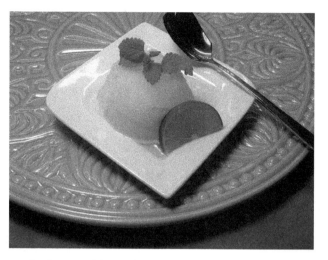

Directions:

1. Freeze ice cream maker tub for about 24 hours before making this sorbet.
2. Add all of the ingredients except the lemon juice in a pan and simmer them over medium heat for about 1 minute or until the sugar dissolves, stirring continuously.
3. Remove the pan from the heat and stir in the lemon juice.
4. Transfer this into an airtight container and refrigerate for about 2 hours.
5. Now, transfer the mixture into an ice cream maker and process it according to the manufacturer's directions.
6. Return the ice cream to the airtight container and freeze for about 2 hours.

Nutrition: Calories 127; Total Fat 0.8 g; Saturated Fat 0.7 g; Cholesterol 0 mg; Sodium 26 mg; Total Carbs 29 g; Fiber 0.6 g; Sugar 25.5 g; Protein 0.8 g

100. Avocado Pudding

Preparation Time: 15 minutes.

Cooking Time: 0 minutes

Servings: 4

Ingredients:

- 2 cups bananas, peeled and chopped
- 2 ripe avocados, peeled, pitted, and chopped
- 1 tsp fresh lime zest, grated finely
- 1 tsp fresh lemon zest, grated finely
- ½ cup fresh lime juice
- ½ cup fresh lemon juice
- 1/3 cup agave nectar

Directions:

1. In a blender, add all the ingredients and pulse until smooth.

2. Transfer the mousse into 4 serving glasses and refrigerate to chill for about 3 hours before serving.

Nutrition: Calories 462; Total Fat 20.1 g; Saturated Fat 4.4 g; Cholesterol 0 mg; Sodium 13 mg; Total Carbs 48.2 g; Fiber 10.2 g; Sugar 30.4 g; Protein 3 g

101. Chocolate Mousse

Preparation Time: 10 minutes.

Cooking Time: 0 minutes

Servings: 4

Ingredients:

- ½ cup unsweetened almond milk
- 1 cup cooked black beans
- 4 Medjool dates, pitted and chopped
- ½ cup pecans, chopped
- 2 tbsp non-alkalized cocoa powder
- 1 tsp organic vanilla extract
- 4 tbsp fresh blueberries

Directions:

1. In a food processor, add all the ingredients and pulse until smooth and creamy.

2. Transfer the mixture into serving bowls and refrigerate to chill before serving.

3. Garnish with blueberries and serve.

Nutrition: Calories 357; Total Fat 13 g; Saturated Fat 1.7 g; Cholesterol 0 mg; Sodium 26 mg; Total Carbs 52.1 g; Fiber 11.9 g; Sugar 16.7 g; Protein 13.4 g

102. Blueberry Crumble

Preparation Time: 15 minutes.

Cooking Time: 40 minutes.

Servings: 4

Ingredients:

- ¼ cup coconut flour
- ¼ cup arrowroot flour
- ¾ tsp baking soda
- ¼ cup ripe banana, peeled and mashed

- 2 tbsp coconut oil, melted
- 3 tbsp filtered water
- ½ tbsp fresh lemon juice
- 1½ cups fresh blueberries

Directions:

1. Prcheat the oven to 300 degrees F. Lightly grease an 8x8-inch baking dish.
2. In a large bowl, add all the ingredients except the blueberries and mix until well combined.
3. In the bottom of the prepared baking dish, place the blueberries and top them with the flour mixture evenly.
4. Bake for about 40 minutes or until the top becomes golden brown.
5. Serve warm.

Nutrition: Calories 107; Total Fat 7.2 g; Saturated Fat 6 g; Cholesterol 0 mg; Sodium 240 mg; Total Carbs 11.6 g; Fiber 2 g; Sugar 6.7 g; Protein 1 g

103. Apple Crisp

Preparation Time: 15 minutes.

Cooking Time: 20 minutes.

Servings: 8

Ingredients:

FOR FILLING:

- 2 large apples, peeled, cored, and chopped
- 2 tbsp water
- 2 tbsp fresh apple juice
- ¼ tsp ground cinnamon

FOR TOPPING:

- ½ cup quick rolled oats
- ¼ cup unsweetened coconut flakes
- 2 tbsp pecans, chopped
- ½ tsp ground cinnamon
- ¼ cup water

Directions:

1. Preheat the oven to 300F. Lightly grease a baking dish.
2. To make the filling add all of the ingredients in a large bowl and gently mix. Set this aside.

3. Make the topping by adding all of the ingredients to another bowl and mix well.
4. Place the filling mixture into the prepared baking dish then spread the topping over the filling mixture evenly.
5. Bake for about 20 minutes or until the top becomes golden brown.
6. Serve warm.

Nutrition: Calories 100; Total Fat 2.7 g; Saturated Fat 0.8 g; Cholesterol 0 mg; Sodium 3 mg; Total Carbs 19.1 g; Fiber 2.6 g; Sugar 11.9 g; Protein 1.2 g

104. Coconut Macaroons

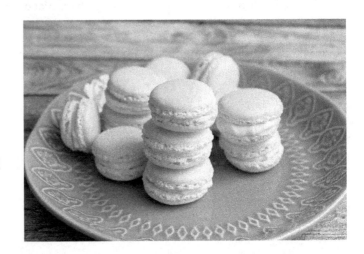

Preparation Time: 15 minutes.

Cooking Time: 10 minutes.

Servings: 12

Ingredients:

- 1½ cups unsweetened coconut, shredded
- 1 tbsp coconut flour
- 1/8 tsp sea salt
- ¼ cup pure maple syrup
- 2 tbsp coconut oil, melted
- 1 tbsp organic vanilla extract

Directions:

1. Preheat the oven to 350 degrees F. Line a large cookie sheet with parchment paper.
2. In a food processor, add all the ingredients and pulse until well combined.
3. Divide the mixture up into tablespoon-size portions and place them onto the prepared cookie sheet in a single layer.
4. Bake for about 7-10 minutes or until golden brown.
5. Remove from the oven and let them cool for about 1 hour before serving.

Nutrition: Calories 78; Total Fat 5.7 g; Saturated Fat 5g; Cholesterol 0 mg; Sodium 22 mg; Total Carbs 6.5 g; Fiber 1.2 g; Sugar 4.7 g; Protein 0.4 g

105. Chickpea Fudge

Preparation Time: 15 minutes.

Cooking Time: 0 minutes

Servings: 12

Ingredients:

- 2 cups cooked chickpeas
- 8 Medjool dates, pitted and chopped
- ½ cup almond butter
- ½ cup unsweetened almond milk
- 1 tsp organic vanilla extract
- 2 tbsp cacao powder

Directions:

1. Line a large baking dish with parchment paper.
2. In a food processor, add all ingredients except the cacao powder and pulse until well combined.
3. Transfer the mixture into a large bowl and stir in the cacao powder.
4. Transfer the mixture onto the prepared baking dish evenly and smooth the surface with a spatula's back.
5. Refrigerate for about 2 hours or until set completely.
6. Cut into desired sized squares and serve.

Nutrition: Calories 172; Total Fat 2.8 g; Saturated Fat 0.3 g; Cholesterol 0 mg; Sodium 16 mg; Total Carbs 32 g; Fiber 7.4 g; Sugar 13 g; Protein 7.1 g

106. Chocolate Crunch Bars

Preparation Time: 5 minutes

Cooking Time: 5 minutes

Servings: 4

Ingredients:

- 1-1/2 cups sugar-free chocolate chips
- 1 cup almond butter
- Stevia to taste
- 1/4 cup coconut oil
- 3 cups pecans, chopped

Directions:

1. Layer an 8-inch baking pan with parchment paper.
2. Mix chocolate chips with butter, coconut oil, and sweetener in a bowl.
3. Melt it by heating in a microwave for 2 to 3 minutes until well mixed.
4. Stir in nuts and seeds. Mix gently.
5. Pour this batter into the baking pan and spread evenly.

6. Refrigerate for 2 to 3 hours.
7. Slice and serve.

Nutrition:

Calories 316; Total Fat 30.9 g; Saturated Fat 8.1 g

Cholesterol 0 mg; Total Carbs 8.3 g; Sugar 1.8 g

Fiber 3.8 g; Sodium 8 mg; Protein 6.4 g

107. Homemade Protein Bar

Preparation Time: 5 minutes

Cooking Time: 10 minutes

Servings: 4

Ingredients:

- 1 cup nut butter
- 4 tablespoons coconut oil
- 2 scoops vanilla protein
- Stevia, to taste
- ½ teaspoon sea salt

OPTIONAL INGREDIENTS:

- 1 teaspoon cinnamon

Directions:

1. Mix coconut oil with butter, protein, stevia, and salt in a dish.
2. Stir in cinnamon and chocolate chip.
3. Press the mixture firmly and freeze until firm.
4. Cut the crust into small bars.
5. Serve and enjoy.

Nutrition:

Calories 179; Total Fat 15.7 g; Saturated Fat 8 g

Cholesterol 0 mg; Total Carbs 4.8 g; Sugar 3.6 g

Fiber 0.8 g; Sodium 43 mg; Protein 5.6 g

108. Shortbread Cookies

Preparation Time: 10 minutes

Cooking Time: 70 minutes

Servings: 6

Ingredients:

- 2 1/2 cups almond flour
- 6 tablespoons nut butter
- 1/2 cup erythritol
- 1 teaspoon vanilla essence

Directions:

1. Preheat your oven to 350 degrees F.
2. Layer a cookie sheet with parchment paper.
3. Beat butter with erythritol until fluffy.
4. Stir in vanilla essence and almond flour. Mix well until becomes crumbly.
5. Spoon out a tablespoon of cookie dough onto the cookie sheet.
6. Add more dough to make as many cookies.
7. Bake for 15 minutes until brown.
8. Serve.

Nutrition: Calories 288; Total Fat 25.3 g

Saturated Fat 6.7 g; Cholesterol 23 mg

Total Carbs 9.6 g; Sugar 0.1 g; Fiber 3.8 g

Sodium 74 mg; Potassium 3 mg; Protein 7.6 g

109. Coconut Chip Cookies

Preparation Time: 10 minutes

Cooking Time: 15 minutes

Servings: 4

Ingredients:

- 1 cup almond flour
- ½ cup cacao nibs
- ½ cup coconut flakes, unsweetened
- 1/3 cup erythritol
- ½ cup almond butter
- ¼ cup nut butter, melted
- ¼ cup almond milk
- Stevia, to taste
- ¼ teaspoon sea salt

Directions:

1. Preheat your oven to 350 degrees F.
2. Layer a cookie sheet with parchment paper.
3. Add and combine all the dry ingredients in a glass bowl.
4. Whisk in butter, almond milk, vanilla essence, stevia, and almond butter.
5. Beat well then stir in dry mixture. Mix well.
6. Spoon out a tablespoon of cookie dough on the cookie sheet.
7. Add more dough to make as many as 16 cookies.
8. Flatten each cookie using your fingers.
9. Bake for 25 minutes until golden brown.
10. Let them sit for 15 minutes.
11. Serve.

Nutrition:

Calories 192; Total Fat 17.44 g; Saturated Fat 11.5 g

Cholesterol 125 mg; Total Carbs 2.2 g; Sugar 1.4 g

Fiber 2.1 g; Sodium 135 mg; Protein 4.7 g

110. Peanut Butter Bars

Preparation Time: 10 minutes

Cooking Time: 10 minutes

Servings: 6

Ingredients:

- 3/4 cup almond flour
- 2 oz. almond butter
- 1/4 cup Swerve
- 1/2 cup peanut butter
- 1/2 teaspoon vanilla

Directions:

1. Combine all the ingredients for bars.
2. Transfer this mixture to 6-inch small pan. Press it firmly.
3. Refrigerate for 30 minutes.
4. Slice and serve.

Nutrition:

Calories 214; Total Fat 19 g; Saturated Fat 5.8 g

Cholesterol 15 mg; Total Carbs 6.5 g; Sugar 1.9 g

Fiber 2.1 g; Sodium 123 mg; Protein 6.5 g

111. Zucchini Bread Pancakes

Preparation Time: 15 minutes

Cooking Time: 35 minutes

Servings: 3

Ingredients:

- Grapeseed oil, 1 tbsp.
- Chopped walnuts, .5 c
- Walnut milk, 2 c
- Shredded zucchini, 1 c
- Mashed burro banana, .25 c
- Date sugar, 2 tbsp.
- Kamut flour or spelt, 2 c

Directions:

1. Place the date sugar and flour into a bowl. Whisk together.
2. Add in the mashed banana and walnut milk. Stir until combined. Remember to scrape the bowl to get all the dry mixture. Add in walnuts and zucchini. Stir well until combined.
3. Place the grapeseed oil onto a griddle and warm.
4. Pour .25 cup batter on the hot griddle. Leave it along until bubbles begin forming on to surface. Carefully turn over the pancake and cook another four minutes until cooked through.
5. Place the pancakes onto a serving plate and enjoy with some agave syrup.

Nutrition:

Calories: 246

Carbohydrates: 49.2 g

Fiber: 4.6 g

Protein: 7.8 g

112. Berry Sorbet

Preparation Time: 10 minutes

Cooking Time: 20 minutes

Servings: 6

Ingredients:

- Water, 2 c
- Blend strawberries, 2 c
- Spelt Flour, 1.5 tsp.

- Date sugar, .5 c

Directions:

1. Pour the water into a large pot and let the water begin to warm. Add the flour and date sugar and stir until dissolved. Allow this mixture to start boiling and continue to cook for around ten minutes. It should have started to thicken. Take off heat and set to the side to cool.

2. Once the syrup has cooled off, add in the strawberries, and stir well to combine.

3. Pour into a container that is freezer safe and put it into the freezer until frozen.

4. Take sorbet out of the freezer, cut into chunks, and put it either into a blender or a food processor. Hit the pulse button until the mixture is creamy.

5. Pour this into the same freezer-safe container and put it back into the freezer for four hours.

Nutrition:

Calories: 99

Carbohydrates: 8 g

Fiber: 3gr

Total Sugar: 2gr

Sodium: 1mg

113. Quinoa Porridge

Preparation Time: 5 minutes

Cooking Time: 15 minutes

Servings: 4

Ingredients:

- Zest of one lime
- Coconut milk, .5 c
- Cloves, .5 tsp.
- Ground ginger, 1.5 tsp.
- Springwater, 2 c
- Quinoa, 1 c
- Grated apple, 1

Directions:

1. Cook the quinoa according to the instructions on the package. When the quinoa has been cooked, drain well. Put it back into the pot and stir in spices.

2. Add coconut milk and stir well to combine.

3. Grate the apple now and stir well.

4. Divide equally into bowls and add the lime zest on top. Sprinkle with nuts and seeds of choice.

Nutrition:

Calories: 180

Fat: 3 g

Carbohydrates: 40 g

Protein: 10 g

114. Apple Quinoa

Preparation Time: 15 minutes

Cooking Time: 30 minutes

Servings: 4

Ingredients:
- Coconut oil, 1 tbsp.
- Ginger
- Key lime .5
- Apple, 1
- Quinoa, .5 c

OPTIONAL TOPPINGS:
- Seeds
- Nuts
- Berries

Directions:

1. Fix the quinoa according to the instructions on the package. When you are getting close to the end of the cooking time, grate in the apple and cook for 30 seconds.
2. Zest the lime into the quinoa and squeeze the juice in. Stir in the coconut oil.
3. Divide evenly into bowls and sprinkle with some ginger.
4. You can add in some berries, nuts, and seeds right before you eat.

Nutrition:

Calories: 779

Fiber: 16.3 g

Fat: 10.3 g

Sodium 12mg

Calcium 101 mg

115. Kamut Porridge

Preparation Time: 10 minutes

Cooking Time: 25 minutes

Servings: 4

Ingredients:
- Agave syrup, 4 tbsp.
- Coconut oil, 1 tbsp.
- Sea salt, .5 tsp.
- Coconut milk, 3.75 c
- Kamut berries, 1 c
- Optional toppings
- Berries
- Coconut chips
- Ground nutmeg
- Ground cloves

Directions:
1. You need to "crack" the Kamut berries. You can do this by placing the berries into a food processor and pulsing until you have 1.25 cups of Kamut.
2. Put the cracked Kamut in a pot with salt and coconut milk. Give it a good stir to combine everything. Allow this mixture to come to a full rolling boil and then turn the heat down until the mixture is simmering. Stir every now and then until the Kamut has thickened to your likeness. This normally takes about ten minutes.
3. Take off heat, stir in agave syrup and coconut oil.
4. Garnish with toppings of choice and enjoy.

Nutrition:

Calories: 114

Protein: 5 g

Carbohydrates: 24g

Fiber: 4 g

116. Hot Kamut With Peaches, Walnuts, And Coconut

Preparation Time: 10 minutes

Cooking Time: 35 minutes

Servings: 4

Ingredients:
- Toasted coconut, 4 tbsp.
- Toasted and chopped walnuts, .5 c
- Chopped dried peaches, 8

- Coconut milk, 3 c
- Kamut cereal, 1 c

Directions:

1. Pour the coconut milk into a saucepan and allow it to warm up. When it begins simmering, add in the Kamut. Let this cook about 15 minutes, while stirring every now and then.

2. When done, divide evenly into bowls and top with the toasted coconut, walnuts, and peaches.

3. You could even go one more and add some fresh berries.

Nutrition:

Calories: 156

Protein: 5.8 g

Carbohydrates: 25 g

Fiber: 6 g

117. Overnight "Oats"

Preparation Time: 5 minutes

Cooking Time: 0 minutes

Servings: 4

Ingredients:

- Berry of choice, .5 c
- Walnut butter, .5 tbsp.
- Burro banana, .5
- Ginger, .5 tsp.
- Coconut milk, .5 c
- Hemp seeds, .5 c

Directions:

1. Put the hemp seeds, salt, and coconut milk into a glass jar. Mix well.

2. Place the lid on the jar and put in the refrigerator to sit overnight.

3. The next morning, add the ginger, berries, and banana. Stir well and enjoy.

Nutrition:

Calories: 139

Fat: 4.1 g

Protein: 9 g

Sugar: 7 g

118. Blueberry Cupcakes

Preparation Time: 15 minutes

Cooking Time: 40 minutes

Servings: 4

Ingredients:
- Grapeseed oil
- Sea salt, .5 tsp.
- Sea moss gel, .25 c
- Agave, .3 c
- Blueberries, .5 c
- Teff flour, .75 c
- Spelt flour, .75 c
- Coconut milk, 1 c

Directions:
1. Warm your oven to 365. Place paper liners into a muffin tin.
2. Place sea moss gel, sea salt, agave, flour, and milk in large bowl. Mix well to combine. Gently fold in blueberries.
3. Gently pour batter into paper liners. Place in oven and bake 30 minutes.
4. They are done when they have turned a nice golden color, and they spring back when you touch them.

Nutrition:

Calories: 85

Fat: 0.7 g

Carbohydrates: 12 g

Protein: 1.4 g

Fiber: 5 g

119. Brazil Nut Cheese

Preparation Time: 2 hours

Cooking Time: 0 minutes

Servings: 4

Ingredients:
- Grapeseed oil, 2 tsp.
- Water, 1.5 c
- Hemp milk, 1.5 c

- Cayenne, .5 tsp.
- Onion powder, 1 tsp.
- Juice of .5 lime
- Sea salt, 2 tsp.
- Brazil nuts, 1 lb.
- Onion powder, 1 tsp.

Directions:

1. You will need to start by soaking the Brazil nuts in some water. You just put the nuts into a bowl and make sure the water covers them. Soak no less than two hours or overnight. Overnight would be best.
2. Now you need to put everything except water into a food processor or blender.
3. Add just .5 cups water and blend for two minutes
4. Continue adding .5 cup water and blending until you have the consistency you want.
5. Scrape into an airtight container and enjoy.

Nutrition:

Calories: 187.

Protein: 4.1 g

Fat: 19 g

Carbs: 3.3 g

Fiber: 2.1

120. Baked Stuffed Pears

Preparation Time: 15 minutes

Cooking Time: 35 minutes

Servings: 4

Ingredients:

- Agave syrup, 4 tbsp.
- Cloves, .25 tsp.
- Chopped walnuts, 4 tbsp.
- Currants, 1 c
- Pears, 4

Directions:

1. Make sure your oven has been warmed to 375.
2. Slice the pears in two lengthwise and remove the core. To get the pear to lay flat, you can slice a small piece off the back side.

3. Place the agave syrup, currants, walnuts, and cloves in a small bowl and mix well. Set this to the side to be used later.

4. Put the pears on a cookie sheet that has parchment paper on it. Make sure the cored sides are facing up. Sprinkle each pear half with about .5 tablespoon of the chopped walnut mixture.

5. Place into the oven and cook for 25 to 30 minutes. Pears should be tender.

Nutrition:

Calories: 103.9

Fiber: 3.1 g

Carbohydrates: 22 g

121. Butternut Squash Pie

Preparation Time: 25 minutes

Cooking Time: 35 minutes

Servings: 4

Ingredients:

FOR THE CRUST

- Cold water
- Agave, splash
- Sea salt, pinch
- Grapeseed oil, .5 c
- Coconut flour, .5 c
- Spelt Flour, 1 c

FOR THE FILLING

- Butternut squash, peeled, chopped
- Water
- Allspice, to taste
- Agave syrup, to taste
- Hemp milk, 1 c
- Sea moss, 4 tbsp.

Directions:

1. You will need to warm your oven to 350.

2. <u>For the Crust:</u> place the grapeseed oil and water into the refrigerator to get it cold. This will take about one hour.

3. Place all ingredients into a large bowl. You need to add in the cold water a little bit in small amounts until a dough form. Place this onto a surface that has been sprinkled with some coconut flour. Knead for a few minutes and roll the dough as thin as you can get it. Carefully pick it up and place it inside a pie plate.

4. Place the butternut squash into a Dutch oven and pour in enough water to cover. Bring this to a full rolling boil. Let this cook until the squash has become soft.

5. Completely drain and place into bowl. Using a potato masher, mash the squash. Add in some allspice and agave to taste. Add in the sea moss and hemp milk. Using a hand mixer, blend well. Pour into the pie crust.

6. Place into the oven and bake for about one hour.

Nutrition:

Calories: 245

Carbohydrates: 50 g

Fat: 10 g

122. Coconut Chia Cream Pot

Preparation Time: 5 minutes

Cooking Time: 5 minutes

Servings: 4

Ingredients:

- Coconut milk (organic), 1 cup
- Coconut yogurt, 1 cup
- Vanilla extract, ½ teaspoon
- Chia seeds, ¼ cup
- Sesame seeds, 1 teaspoon
- Flaxseed (ground), 1 tablespoon or flax meal, 1 tablespoon

TOPPINGS:

- Blueberries, 1 handful
- Mixed nuts (brazil nuts, almonds, pistachios, macadamia, etc.)
- Cinnamon (ground), one teaspoon

Directions:

1. First, blend the date with coconut milk (the idea is to sweeten the coconut milk).

2. Get a mixing bowl and add the coconut milk with the vanilla, sesame seeds, chia seeds, and flax meal.

3. Refrigerate for between twenty to thirty minutes or wait till the chia expands.

4. To serve, pour a layer of coconut yogurt in a small glass, then add the chia mix, followed by pouring another layer of the coconut yogurt. It's alkaline, creamy and delicious!

Nutrition:

Calories: 310

Carbohydrates: 39 g

Protein: 4 g

Fiber: 8.1 g

123. Chocolate Avocado Mousse

Preparation Time: 10 minutes

Cooking Time: 5 minutes

Servings: 4

Ingredients:

- Coconut water, 2/3 cup
- Avocado, ½ hass
- Raw cacao, 2 teaspoons
- Vanilla, 1 teaspoon
- Dates, 3
- Sea salt, 1 teaspoon
- Dark chocolate shavings

Directions:

1. Add all ingredients in a food processor or blender.

2. Blast until it becomes thick and smooth, as you wish.

3. Put in a fridge and allow it to get firm.

Nutrition:

Calories: 185

Fat: 12.6 gr

Protein: 2.1 g

Carbohydrate: 16.9 gr

Calcium: 17 mg

124. Chia Vanilla Coconut Pudding

Preparation Time: 5 minutes

Cooking Time: 5 minutes

Servings: 2

Ingredients:

- Coconut oil, 2 tablespoons
- Raw cashew, ½ cup
- Coconut water, ½ cup
- Cinnamon, 1 teaspoon
- Dates (pitted), 3
- Vanilla, 2 teaspoons
- Coconut flakes (unsweetened), 1 teaspoon
- Salt (Himalayan or Celtic Grey)
- Chia seeds, 6 tablespoons
- Cinnamon or pomegranate seeds for garnish (optional)

Directions:

1. Get a blender, add all the ingredients (minus the pomegranate and chia seeds), and blend for about forty to sixty seconds.
2. Reduce the blender speed to the lowest and add the chia seeds.
3. Pour the content into an airtight container and put in a refrigerator for five to six hours.
4. To serve, you can garnish with the cinnamon powder of pomegranate seeds.

Nutrition:

Calories: 201

Fat: 10 g

Sodium: 32.8 mg

Sugar: 8 gr

125. Sweet Tahini Dip With Ginger Cinnamon Fruit

Preparation Time: 10 minutes

Cooking Time: 5 minutes

Servings: 2

Ingredients:

- Cinnamon, 1 teaspoon
- Green apple, 1
- Pear, 1
- Fresh ginger, 2 or 3

- Celtic sea salt, 1 teaspoon
- Ingredient for sweet Tahini
- Almond butter (raw), 3 teaspoons
- Tahini (one big scoop), 3 teaspoons
- Coconut oil, 2 teaspoons
- Cayenne (optional), ¼ teaspoons
- Wheat-free tamari, 2 teaspoons
- Liquid coconut nectar, 1 teaspoon

Directions:

1. Get a clean mixing bowl.
2. Grate the ginger, add cinnamon, sea salt and mix together in the bowl.
3. Dice apple and pear into little cubes, turn into the bowl and mix.
4. Get a mixing bowl and mix all the ingredients.
5. Then add the Sprinkle the Sweet Tahini Dip all over the Ginger Cinnamon Fruit.
6. Serve.

Nutrition:

Calories: 109

Fat: 10.8 g

Sodium: 258 mg

Fiber: 24.7 g

126. Coconut Butter And Chopped Berries With Mint

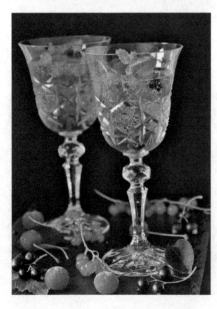

Preparation Time: 5 minutes

Cooking Time: 5 minutes

Servings: 04

Ingredients:

- Chopped mint, 1 tablespoon
- Coconut butter (melted), 2 tablespoons
- Mixed berries (strawberries, blueberries, and raspberries)

Directions:

1. Get a small bowl and add the berries.
2. Drizzle the melted coconut butter and sprinkle the mint.
3. Serve.

Nutrition: Calories: 159 - Fat: 12 g - Carbohydrates: 18 g

127. Alkaline Raw Pumpkin Pie

Preparation Time: 5 minutes

Cooking Time: 5 minutes

Servings: 4

Ingredients:

FOR PIE CRUST

- Cinnamon, 1 teaspoon
- Dates/Turkish apricots, 1 cup
- Raw almonds, 1 cup
- Coconut flakes (unsweetened), 1 cup

FOR PIE FILLING

- Dates, 6
- Cinnamon, ½ teaspoon
- Nutmeg, ½ teaspoon
- Pecans (soaked overnight), 1 cup
- Organic pumpkin Blends (12 oz.), 1 ¼ cup
- Nutmeg, ½ teaspoon
- Sea salt (Himalayan or Celtic Sea Salt), ¼ teaspoon
- Vanilla, 1 teaspoon
- Gluten-free tamari

Directions:

Directions for pie crust:

1. Get a food processor and blend all the pie crust ingredients at the same time.
2. Make sure the mixture turns oily and sticky before you stop mixing.
3. Place the mixture in a pie pan and mold against the sides and floor, to make itstic properly.

Directions for the pie filling:

4. Blend all the ingredients together in a blender.
5. Add mixture to fill in the pie crust.
6. Pour some cinnamon on top.
7. Then refrigerate till it's cold. Then mold.

Nutrition:

Calories 135

Calories from Fat 41.4.

Total Fat 4.6 g

Cholesterol 11.3 mg

128. Strawberry Sorbet

Preparation Time: 5 minutes

Cooking Time: 4 Hours

Servings: 4

Ingredients:

- 2 cups of Strawberries
- 1 1/2 teaspoons of Spelt Flour
- 1/2 cup of Date Sugar
- 2 cups of Spring Water

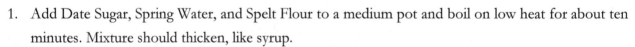

Directions:

1. Add Date Sugar, Spring Water, and Spelt Flour to a medium pot and boil on low heat for about ten minutes. Mixture should thicken, like syrup.
2. Remove the pot from the heat and allow it to cool.
3. After cooling, add Blend Strawberry and mix gently.
4. Put this mixture in a container and freeze.
5. Cut it into pieces, put the sorbet into a processor and blend until smooth.
6. Put everything back in the container and leave in the refrigerator for at least four hours.
7. Serve and enjoy your Strawberry Sorbet!

Nutrition:

Calories: 120

Carbohydrates: 31 g

Sodium: 1 mg

Fiber: 1.6 gr

Sugar: 28.5 gr

129. Blueberry Muffins

Preparation Time: 5 minutes

Cooking Time: 1 Hour

Servings: 3

Ingredients:

- 1/2 cup of Blueberries
- 3/4 cup of Teff Flour
- 3/4 cup of Spelt Flour
- 1/3 cup of Agave Syrup
- 1/2 teaspoon of Pure Sea Salt
- 1 cup of Coconut Milk
- 1/4 cup of Sea Moss Gel (optional)
- Grape Seed Oil

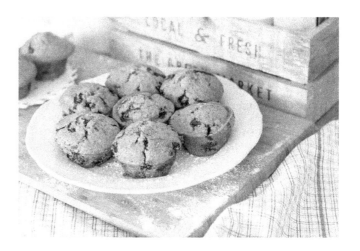

Directions:

1. Preheat your oven to 365 degrees Fahrenheit.
2. Grease or line 6 standard muffin cups.
3. Add Teff, Spelt flour, Pure Sea Salt, Coconut Milk, Sea Moss Gel, and Agave Syrup to a large bowl. Mix them together.
4. Add Blueberries to the mixture and mix well.
5. Divide muffin batter among the 6 muffin cups.
6. Bake for 30 minutes until golden brown.
7. Serve and enjoy your Blueberry Muffins!

Nutrition: Calories: 65

Fat: 0.7 g

Carbohydrates: 12 g

Protein: 1.4 g

Fiber: 5 g

130. Banana Strawberry Ice Cream

Preparation Time: 5 minutes

Cooking Time: 4 Hours

Servings: 5

Ingredients:

- 1 cup of Strawberry
- 5 quartered Baby Bananas
- 1/2 Avocado, chopped
- 1 tablespoon of Agave Syrup
- 1/4 cup of Homemade Walnut Milk

Directions:

1. Put all ingredients into the blender and blend them well.
2. Taste. If it is too thick, add extra Milk or Agave Syrup if you want it sweeter.
3. Place in a container with a lid and allow to freeze for at least 5 to 6 hours.
4. Serve it and enjoy your Banana Strawberry Ice Cream!

Nutrition:

Calories: 200

Fat: 10.5 g

Sodium: 6 mg

Carbohydrates: 34 g

Calcium: 14 mg

131. Homemade Whipped Cream

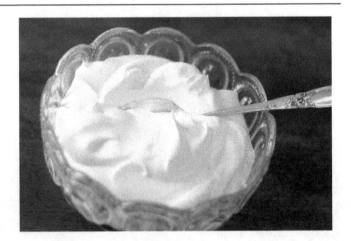

Preparation Time: 5 minutes

Cooking Time: 10 Minutes

Servings: 1 Cup

Ingredients:

*   1 cup of Aquafaba
*   1/4 cup of Agave Syrup

Directions:

1. Add Agave Syrup and Aquafaba into a bowl.
2. Mix at high speed around 5 minutes with a stand mixer or 10 to 15 minutes with a hand mixer.
3. Serve and enjoy your Homemade Whipped Cream!

Nutrition:

Calories: 21

Fat: 0g

Sodium: 0.3g

Carbohydrates: 5.3g

Fiber: 0g

Sugars: 4.7g

Protein: 0g

Snack Recipes

132. Pumpkin spice crackers

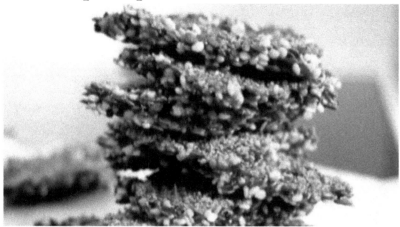

Preparation Time: 10 minutes

Cooking Time: 60 minutes

Servings: 6

Ingredients:

- 1/3 cup coconut flour
- 2 tablespoons pumpkin pie spice
- ¾ cup sunflower seeds
- ¾ cup flaxseed
- 1/3 cup sesame seeds
- 1 tablespoon ground psyllium husk powder
- 1 teaspoon sea salt
- 3 tablespoons coconut oil, melted
- 1 1/3 cups alkaline water

Directions:

1. Set your oven to 300 degrees F.
2. Combine all dry ingredients in a bowl.
3. Add water and oil to the mixture and mix well.
4. Let the dough stay for 2 to 3 mins.
5. Spread the dough on a cookie sheet lined with parchment paper.
6. Bake for 30 minutes.
7. Reduce the oven heat to low and bake for another 30 minutes.

8. Crack the bread into bite-size pieces.

9. Serve

Nutrition:

Calories 248; Total Fat 15.7 g; Saturated Fat 2.7 g

Cholesterol 75 mg; Sodium 94 mg; Total Carbs 0.4 g

Fiber 0g; Sugar 0 g; Protein 24.9 g

133. Spicy roasted nuts

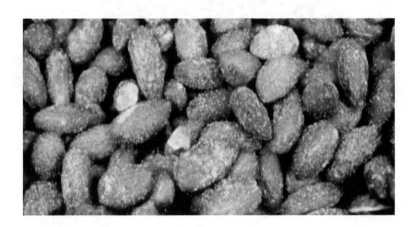

Nutrition:

Calories 287; Total Fat 29.5 g;

Saturated Fat 3 g; Cholesterol 0 mg;

Total Carbs 5.9 g; Sugar 1.4g

Fiber 4.3 g; Sodium 388 mg;

Protein 4.2 g

Preparation Time: 10 minutes

Cooking Time: 15 minutes

Servings: 4

Ingredients:

- 8 oz. pecans or almonds or walnuts
- 1 teaspoon sea salt
- 1 tablespoon olive oil or coconut oil
- 1 teaspoon ground cumin
- 1 teaspoon paprika powder or chili powder

Directions:

1. Add all the ingredients to a skillet.

2. Roast the nuts until golden brown.

3. Serve and enjoy.

134. Wheat Crackers

Preparation Time: 10 minutes

Cooking Time: 20 minutes

Servings: 4

Ingredients:

- 1 3/4 cups almond flour

- 1 1/2 cups coconut flour
- 3/4 teaspoon sea salt
- 1/3 cup vegetable oil
- 1 cup alkaline water
- Sea salt for sprinkling

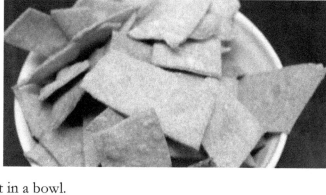

Directions:

1. Set your oven to 350 degrees F.
2. Mix coconut flour, almond flour and salt in a bowl.
3. Stir in vegetable oil and water. Mix well until smooth.
4. Spread this dough on a floured surface into a thin sheet.
5. Cut small squares out of this sheet.
6. Arrange the dough squares on a baking sheet lined with parchment paper.
7. Bake for 20 minutes until light golden in color.
8. Serve.

Nutrition:

Calories 64; Total Fat 9.2 g; Saturated Fat 2.4 g

Cholesterol 110 mg; Sodium 276 mg; Total Carbs 9.2 g;

Fiber 0.9 g; Sugar 1.4 g; Protein 1.5 g

135. Potato Chips

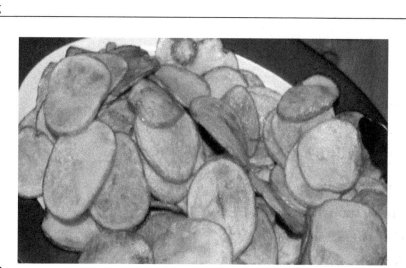

Preparation Time: 10 minutes

Cooking Time: 5 minutes

Servings: 4

Ingredients:

- 1 tablespoon vegetable oil
- 1 potato, sliced paper thin
- Sea salt, to taste

Directions:

1. Toss potato with oil and sea salt.
2. Spread the slices in a baking dish in a single layer.
3. Cook in a microwave for 5 minutes until golden brown.
4. Serve.

Nutrition: Calories 80

Total Fat 3.5 g; Saturated Fat 0.1 g; Cholesterol 320 mg; Sugar 0.7 g

Sodium 350 mg; Total Carbs 11.6 g; Fiber 0.7 g; Protein 1.2 g

136. Zucchini Pepper Chips

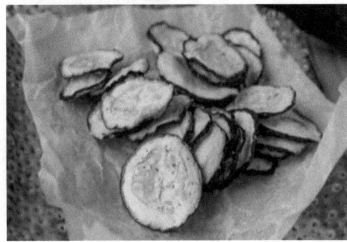

Preparation Time: 10 minutes

Cooking Time: 15 minutes

Servings: 4

Ingredients:

- 1 2/3 cups vegetable oil
- 1 teaspoon garlic powder
- 1 teaspoon onion powder
- 1/2 teaspoon black pepper
- 3 tablespoons crushed red pepper flakes
- 2 zucchinis, thinly sliced

Directions:

1. Mix oil with all the spices in a bowl.
2. Add zucchini slices and mix well.
3. Transfer the mixture to a Ziplock bag and seal it.
4. Refrigerate for 10 minutes.
5. Spread the zucchini slices on a greased baking sheet.
6. Bake for 15 minutes
7. Serve.

Nutrition:

Calories 172; Total Fat 11.1 g; Saturated Fat 5.8 g; Sugar 0.2 g; Protein 13.5 g

Cholesterol 610 mg; Sodium 749 mg; Total Carbs 19.9 g; Fiber 0.2 g

137. Apple Chips

Preparation Time: 5 minutes

Cooking Time: 45 minutes

Servings: 4

Ingredients:

- 2 Golden Delicious apples, cored and thinly sliced
- 1 ½ teaspoons white sugar
- ½ teaspoon ground cinnamon

Directions:

1. Set your oven to 225 degrees F.
2. Place apple slices on a baking sheet.
3. Sprinkle sugar on it.
4. Add cinnamon over apple slices.
5. Bake for 45 minutes.
6. Serve.

Nutrition:

Calories 127; Total Fat 3.5 g;

Saturated Fat 0.5 g; Cholesterol 162 mg;

Sodium 142 mg; Total Carbs 33.6g

Fiber 0.4 g; Sugar 0.5 g; Protein 4.5 g

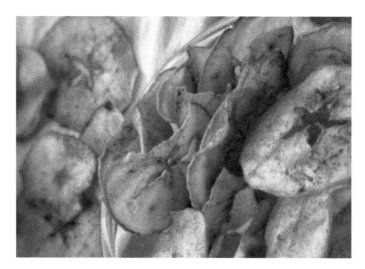

138. Carrot Chips

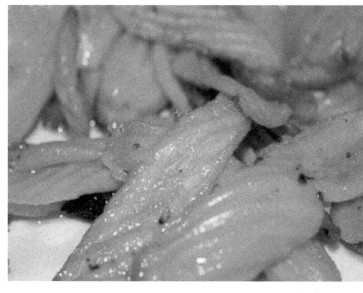

Nutrition:

Calories 153; Total Fat 7.5 g;

Saturated Fat 1.1 g; Cholesterol 20 mg;

Sodium 97 mg; Total Carbs 20.4 g

Fiber 0 g; Sugar 0 g; Protein 3.1g

Preparation Time: 5 minutes

Cooking Time: 12 minutes

Servings: 4

Ingredients:

- 4 carrots, washed, peeled and sliced
- 2 teaspoons extra-virgin olive oil
- 1/4 teaspoon sea salt

Directions:

1. Set your oven to 350 degrees F.
2. Toss carrots with salt and olive oil.
3. Spread the slices on two baking sheets in a single layer.
4. Bake for 6 minutes on upper and lower rack of the oven.
5. Switch the baking racks and bake for another 6 minutes.
6. Serve.

139. Pita Chips

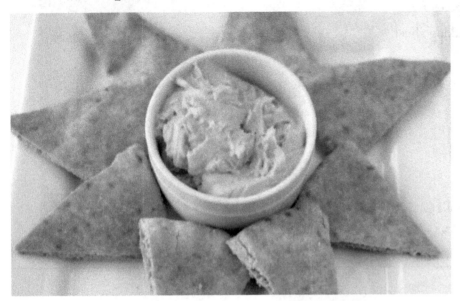

Preparation Time: 5 minutes

Cooking Time: 7 minutes

Servings: 4

Ingredients:

- 12 pita bread pockets, sliced into triangles
- 1/2 cup olive oil
- 1/2 teaspoon ground black pepper
- 1 teaspoon garlic salt
- 1/2 teaspoon dried basil
- 1 teaspoon dried chervil

Directions:

1. Set your oven to 400 degrees F.
2. Toss pita with all the remaining ingredients in a bowl.
3. Spread the seasoned triangles on a baking sheet.
4. Bake for 7 minutes until golden brown.
5. Serve with your favorite hummus.

Nutrition:

Calories 201; Total Fat 5.5 g; Saturated Fat 2.1 g

Cholesterol 10 mg; Sodium 597 mg; Total Carbs 2.4 g

Fiber 0 g; Sugar 0 g; Protein 3.1g

140. Sweet Potato Chips

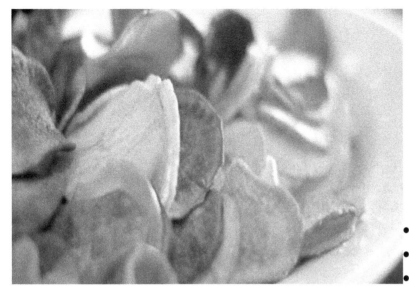

Nutrition:

Calories 213; Cholesterol 120 mg;
Total Fat 8.5g; Saturated Fat 3.1g;
Sodium 497mg; Total Carbs 21.4g
Fiber 0g; Sugar 0g; Protein 0.1g

Preparation Time: 5 minutes

Cooking Time: 5 minutes

Servings: 4

Ingredients:

- 1 sweet potato, thinly sliced
- 2 teaspoons olive oil, or as needed
- Coarse sea salt, to taste

Directions:

1. Toss sweet potato with oil and salt.
2. Spread the slices in a baking dish in a single layer.
3. Cook in a microwave for 5 minutes until golden brown.
4. Serve.

141. Chocolate Milkshake

Preparation Time: 10 minutes

Cooking Time: 0 minutes.

Servings: 2

Ingredients:

- 2 large frozen bananas, peeled
- 1 tbsp almond butter
- 1 tbsp cacao powder
- ¼ tsp organic vanilla extract
- 1½ cups unsweetened almond milk

Directions:

1. Add all the ingredients in a high-speed blender and pulse until smooth.
2. Pour the milkshake into two glasses and serve immediately.

Nutrition: Calories 208; Total Fat 8.1 g; Saturated Fat 1 g; Cholesterol 0 mg; Sodium 137 mg; Total Carbs 35.4 g; Fiber 5.8 g; Sugar 17.1 g; Protein 4.4 g

142. Strawberry Gazpacho

Preparation Time: 15 minutes.

Cooking Time: 0 minutes

Servings: 4

Ingredients:

- 1½ lbs fresh strawberries, hulled and sliced plus more for garnishing
- ½ cup red bell pepper, seeded and chopped
- 1 small cucumber, peeled, seeded, and chopped
- ¼ cup onion, chopped
- ¼ cup fresh basil leaves
- 1 small garlic clove, chopped
- ¼ small jalapeño pepper, seeded and chopped
- 1 tbsp olive oil
- 3 tbsp balsamic vinegar

Directions:

1. In a high-seed blender, add 1½ pounds of the strawberries and the remaining ingredients and pulse until well combined and smooth.
2. Transfer the gazpacho into a large serving bowl.
3. Cover the bowl and refrigerate to chill completely before serving.
4. Serve chilled garnished with extra strawberry slices.

Nutrition: Calories 107; Total Fat 4.2 g; Saturated Fat 0.5 g; Cholesterol 0 mg; Sodium 5 mg; Total Carbs 17.8 g; Fiber 4.2 g; Sugar 10.8 g; Protein 1.1 g

143. Tomato Salsa

Preparation Time: 15 minutes.

Cooking Time: 0 minutes

Servings: 4

Ingredients:

- 3 large tomatoes, chopped
- 1 small red onion, chopped
- ¼ cup fresh cilantro leaves, chopped

- 1 jalapeño pepper, seeded and chopped finely
- 1 small garlic clove, minced finely
- 2 tbsp fresh lime juice
- 1 tbsp extra-virgin olive oil
- Sea salt and freshly ground black pepper, to taste

Directions:

1. In a large bowl, add all the ingredients and gently toss to coat well.
2. Serve immediately.

Nutrition: Calories 64; Total Fat 3.8 g; Saturated Fat 0.5 g; Cholesterol 0 mg; Sodium 66 mg; Total Carbs 7.5 g; Fiber 2.2 g; Sugar 4.5 g; Protein 15 g

144. Avocado Guacamole

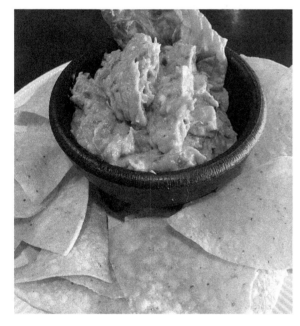

Preparation Time: 10 minutes.

Cooking Time: 0 minutes

Servings: 4

Ingredients:

- 2 medium ripe avocados, peeled, pitted, and chopped
- 1 small red onion, chopped
- 1 garlic clove, minced
- 1 Serrano pepper, seeded and chopped
- 1 tomato, seeded and chopped
- 2 tbsp fresh cilantro leaves, chopped
- 1 tbsp fresh lime juice
- Sea salt, to taste

Directions:

1. In a large bowl, add avocado and mash it completely with a fork.
2. Add the remaining ingredients and gently stir to combine.
3. Serve immediately.

Nutrition: Calories 217; Total Fat 19.7 g; Saturated Fat 4.1 g; Cholesterol 0 mg; Sodium 67 mg; Total Carbs 11.3 g; Fiber 7.4 g; Sugar 1.7 g; Protein 2.3 g

145. Cauliflower Hummus

Preparation Time: 15 minutes.

Cooking Time: 5 minutes.

Servings: 6

Ingredients:

- 1 medium head cauliflower, trimmed and chopped
- 2 garlic cloves, chopped
- 2 tbsp almond butter
- 2 tbsp olive oil
- Sea salt, to taste
- 2 tbsp fresh chives, minced
- Pinch of cayenne pepper

Directions:

1. A large pan of boiling water adds the cauliflower and cook over medium heat for about 4-5 minutes.
2. Remove from the heat and drain the cauliflower well.
3. Set aside to cool it slightly.
4. In a food processor, add the cauliflower, garlic, almond butter, oil, salt, and pulse until smooth.
5. Transfer the hummus into a serving bowl.
6. Sprinkle with chives and cayenne pepper and serve immediately.

Nutrition: Calories 103; Total Fat 9.3 g; Saturated Fat 1.1 g; Cholesterol 0 mg; Sodium 63 mg; Total Carbs 4.5 g; Fiber 2 g; Sugar 1.6 g; Protein 2.5 g

146. Kale Chips

Preparation Time: 10 minutes.

Cooking Time: 15 minutes

Servings: 6

Ingredients:

- 1 lb fresh kale leaves, stemmed and torn
- ¼ tsp cayenne pepper
- Sea salt, to taste
- 1 tbsp olive oil

Directions:

1. Preheat oven to 350 degrees F. Line a large baking sheet with parchment paper.
2. Arrange the kale pieces onto the prepared baking sheet in a single layer.
3. Sprinkle the kale with cayenne pepper and salt and drizzle with oil.

4. Bake for about 10-15 minutes.
5. Remove from the oven and let it cool before serving.

Nutrition: Calories 57; Total Fat 2.3 g; Saturated Fat 0.3 g; Cholesterol 0 mg; Sodium 72 mg; Total Carbs 8 g; Fiber 1.2 g; Sugar 0 g; Protein 2.3 g

147. Sweet Potato Fries

Preparation Time: 10 minutes.

Cooking Time: 25 minutes

Servings: 2

Ingredients:

- 1 large sweet potato, peeled and cut into wedges
- 1 tsp ground turmeric
- 1 tsp ground cinnamon
- Sea salt and freshly ground black pepper, to taste
- 2 tbsp extra-virgin olive oil

Directions:

1. Preheat the oven to 425 degrees F. Line a baking sheet with a piece of foil.
2. In a large bowl, add all ingredients and toss to coat well.
3. Transfer the potatoes onto the prepared baking sheet and spread into an even layer.
4. Bake for about 25 minutes, flipping once after 15 minutes.
5. Remove from the oven and serve immediately.

Nutrition: Calories 199; Total Fat 14.3 g; Saturated Fat 2 g; Cholesterol 0 mg; Sodium 146 mg; Total Carbs 18.2 g; Fiber 3.5 g; Sugar 5.3 g; Protein 1.8 g

148. Seed Crackers

Preparation Time: 15 minutes.

Cooking Time: 20 minutes.

Servings: 6

Ingredients:

- 3 tbsp water
- 1 tbsp chia seeds
- 3 tbsp sunflower seeds
- 1 tbsp quinoa flour
- 1 tsp ground turmeric

- Pinch of ground cinnamon
- Salt, to taste

Directions:

1. Preheat the oven to 345 degrees F. Line a baking sheet with parchment paper.
2. In a bowl, add the water and chia seeds and soak them for about 15 minutes.
3. After 15 minutes, add the remaining ingredients and mix well.
4. Spread the mixture onto the prepared baking sheet.
5. With a pizza cutter, cut the formed mixture into desired shapes.
6. Bake for about 20 minutes.
7. Remove from the oven and place it onto a wire rack to cool completely before serving.

Nutrition: Calories 26; Total Fat 1.6 g; Saturated Fat 0.1 g; Cholesterol 0 mg; Sodium 28 mg; Total Carbs 2.5 g; Fiber 1.3 g; Sugar 0.1 g; Protein 1 g

149. Veggie Bites

Preparation Time: 20 minutes.

Cooking Time: 40 minutes.

Servings: 6

Ingredients:

- 2 medium sweet potatoes, peeled and cubed into ½-inch chunks
- 2 tbsp coconut milk
- 1 cup fresh kale leaves, trimmed and chopped
- 1 medium shallot, chopped finely
- 1 tsp ground cumin
- ½ tsp granulated garlic
- ¼ tsp ground turmeric
- Sea salt and freshly ground black pepper, to taste
- Ground flax seeds, as needed

Directions:

1. Preheat the oven to 400 degrees F. Line a baking sheet with parchment paper.
2. Arrange a steamer basket in a pot of water.
3. Place the sweet potatoes in the steamer basket and steam for about 10-15 minutes.
4. Place the sweet potatoes and coconut milk in a large bowl and mash them well with a potato masher.
5. Add the remaining ingredients except flax seeds and mix until well combined.

6. Make about 1½-2-inch balls from the mixture.
7. Arrange the balls onto the prepared baking sheet in a single layer and sprinkle with the flax seeds.
8. Bake for about 20-25 minutes.
9. Remove from the oven and serve warm.

Nutrition: Calories 135; Total Fat 4.3 g; Saturated Fat 1.5 g; Cholesterol 0 mg; Sodium 41 mg; Total Carbs 20.2 g; Fiber 5.3 g; Sugar 1.4 g; Protein 3.3 g

150. Roasted Pumpkin Seeds

Preparation Time: 10 minutes.

Cooking Time: 20 minutes.

Servings: 4

Ingredients:

- 1 cup pumpkin seeds, washed and dried
- 2 tsp garam masala
- 1/3 tsp red chili powder
- ¼ tsp ground turmeric
- Sea salt, to taste
- 3 tbsp coconut oil, meted
- ½ tbsp fresh lemon juice

Directions:

1. Preheat the oven to 350 degrees F.
2. Add all ingredients except lemon juice to a bowl and toss to coat well.
3. Transfer the pumpkin seed mixture onto a baking sheet.
4. Roast for about 20 minutes, flipping occasionally.
5. Remove from oven and set aside to cool completely before serving.
6. Drizzle with the lemon juice and serve.

Nutrition: Calories 276; Total Fat 26.1 g; Saturated Fat 11.8 g; Cholesterol 0 mg; Sodium 69 mg; Total Carbs 6.4 g; Fiber 1.5 g; Sugar 0.4 g; Protein 8.6 g

151. Bean Burgers

Preparation Time: 20 minutes

Cooking Time: 25 minutes

Servings: 8

Ingredients:

- ½ cup walnuts
- 1 carrot, peeled and chopped
- 1 celery stalk, chopped
- 4 scallions, chopped
- 5 garlic cloves, chopped
- 2¼ cups canned black beans, rinsed and drained
- 2½ cups sweet potato, peeled and grated
- ½ teaspoon red pepper flakes, crushed
- ¼ teaspoon cayenne pepper
- Sea salt and freshly ground black pepper, to taste

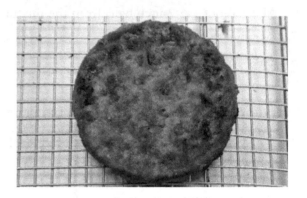

Directions:

1. Preheat the oven to 400 degrees F. Line a baking sheet with parchment paper.
2. In a food processor, add the walnuts and pulse until finely ground.
3. Add the carrot, celery, scallion, and garlic and pulse until chopped finely.
4. Transfer the vegetable mixture into a large bowl.
5. In the same food processor, add the beans and pulse until chopped.
6. Add 1½ cups of the sweet potato and pulse until a chunky mixture form.
7. Transfer the bean mixture into the bowl with the vegetable mixture.
8. Stir in remaining sweet potato and spices and mix until well combined.
9. Make 8 equal sized patties from the mixture.
10. Arrange the patties onto the prepared baking sheet in a single layer.
11. Bake for about 25 minutes.
12. Serve hot.

Nutrition:

Calories 300; Total Fat 5.5 g; Saturated Fat 0.5 g Cholesterol 0 mg; Sodium 65 mg; Total Carbs 49.8 g Fiber 11.4g; Sugar 5.9 g; Protein 15.3 g

152. Grilled Watermelon

Preparation Time: 10 minutes

Cooking Time: 4 minutes

Servings: 4

Ingredients:

- 1 watermelon, peeled and cut into 1-inch thick wedges

- 1 garlic clove, minced finely
- 2 tablespoons fresh lime juice
- Pinch of cayenne pepper
- Pinch of sea salt

Directions:

1. Preheat the grill to high heat. Grease the grill grate.
2. Grill the watermelon pieces for about 2 minutes on both sides.
3. Meanwhile, in a small bowl mix together the remaining ingredients.
4. Drizzle the watermelon slices with the lemon mixture and serve.

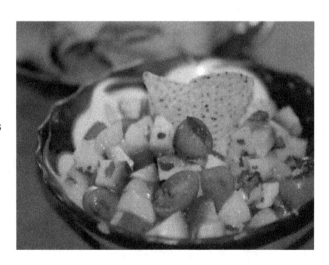

Nutrition:

Calories 11; Total Fat 0.1 g; Saturated Fat 0 g

Cholesterol 0 mg; Sodium 59 mg; Total Carbs 2.6 g

Fiber 0.2 g; Sugar 1.9 g; Protein 0.2 g

---

153. Mango Salsa

Preparation Time: 15 minutes

Cooking Time: 15 minutes

Servings: 6

Ingredients:

- 1 avocado, peeled, pitted, and cut into cubes
- 2 tablespoons fresh lime juice
- 1 mango, peeled, pitted, and cubed
- 1 cup cherry tomatoes, halved
- 1 jalapeño pepper, seeded and chopped
- 1 tablespoon fresh cilantro, chopped
- Sea salt, to taste

Directions:

1. In a large bowl, add the avocado and lime juice and mix well.
2. Add the remaining ingredients and stir to combine.
3. Serve immediately.

154. Avocado Gazpacho

Preparation Time: 15 minutes

Cooking Time: 0 minutes

Servings: 6

Ingredients:

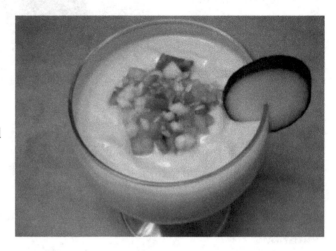

- 3 large avocados, peeled, pitted, and chopped
- 1/3 cup fresh cilantro leaves
- 3 cups homemade vegetable broth
- 2 tablespoons fresh lemon juice
- 1 teaspoon ground cumin
- ¼ teaspoon cayenne pepper
- Sea salt, to taste

Directions:

1. Add all the ingredients in a high-speed blender and pulse until smooth.
2. Transfer the soup into a large bowl.
3. Cover the bowl and refrigerate to chill for at least 2-3 hours before serving.

Nutrition:

Calories 227 - Total Fat 20.4 g - Saturated Fat 4.4 g - Cholesterol 0 mg - Sodium 429 mg Total Carbs 9.4 g - Fiber 6.8 g - Sugar 1 g - Protein 4.5 g

155. Roasted Chickpeas

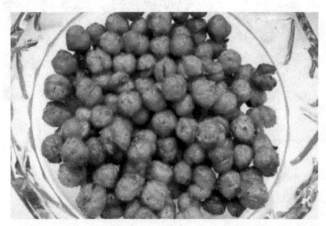

Preparation Time: 10 minutes

Cooking Time: 45 minutes

Servings: 12

Ingredients:

- 4 cups cooked chickpeas
- ¼ teaspoon ground cumin
- 2 garlic cloves, minced
- ½ teaspoon smoked paprika
- ½ teaspoon dried oregano, crushed

- salt, to taste
- 1 tablespoon olive oil

Directions:

1. Preheat the oven to 400 degrees F. Grease a large baking sheet.
2. Place chickpeas onto the prepared baking sheet in a single layer.
3. Roast for about 30 minutes, stirring the chickpeas every 10 minutes.
4. Meanwhile, in a small mixing bowl, mix together garlic, thyme, and spices.
5. Remove the baking sheet from the oven.
6. Pour the garlic mixture and oil over the chickpeas and toss to coat well.
7. Roast for about 10-15 minutes more.
8. Now, turn the oven off but leave the baking sheet inside for about 10 minutes before serving.

Nutrition:

Calories 92 - Total Fat 1.9 g - Saturated Fat 0.2 g - Cholesterol 0 mg - Sodium 166 mg - Total Carbs 15 g Fiber 0.1 g - Sugar 4 g - Protein 4.1 g

156. Banana Chips

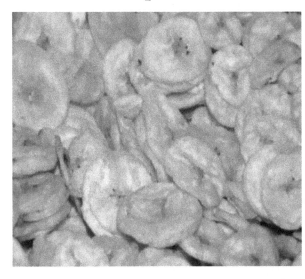

Nutrition:

Calories 61; Total Fat 0.2 g; Saturated Fat 0.1 g

Cholesterol 0 mg; Sodium 1 mg;

Total Carbs 15.5 g; Fiber 1.8 g;

Sugar 8.3 g; Protein 0.7 g

Preparation Time: 10 minutes

Cooking Time: 1 hour

Servings: 4

Ingredients:

- 2 large bananas, peeled and cut into ¼-inch thick slices

Directions:

1. Prepare the oven to 250 degrees F. Line a large baking sheet with baking paper.
2. Place the banana slices onto the prepared baking sheet in a single layer.
3. Bake for about 1 hour.

157. Roasted Cashews

Preparation Time: 10 minutes

Cooking Time: 10 minutes

Servings: 12

Ingredients:

- 2 cups raw cashews
- ½ teaspoon ground cumin
- ¼ teaspoon cayenne pepper
- Pinch of salt
- 1 tablespoon fresh lemon juice

Directions:

1. Preheat the oven to 400 degrees F. Line a large roasting pan with a piece of foil.
2. In a large bowl, add the cashews and spices and toss to coat well.
3. Transfer the cashews to the prepared roasting pan.
4. Roast for about 8-10 minutes.
5. Drizzle with lemon juice and serve.

Nutrition:

Calories 132 - Total Fat 10.6g - Saturated Fat 2.1g - Cholesterol 0mg - Sodium 16mg - Total Carbs 7.6g
Fiber 0.7 g - Sugar 1.2 g - Protein 3.5 g

158. Dried Orange Slices

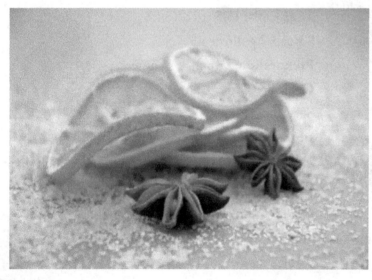

Nutrition:

Calories 23; Total Fat 0.1 g;
Saturated Fat 0 g; Cholesterol 0 mg;
Sodium 0 mg; Total Carbs 5.8 g
Fiber 3.5 g; Sugar 4.6 g; Protein 0.5 g

Preparation Time: 10 minutes

Cooking Time: 1 hours

Servings: 15

Ingredients:

- 4 seedless navel oranges, cut into thin slices (do NOT peel oranges)

Directions:

1. Set the dehydrator to 135 degrees F.
2. Arrange the orange slices onto the dehydrator sheets.
3. Dehydrate for about 10 hours.

159. Chickpea Hummus

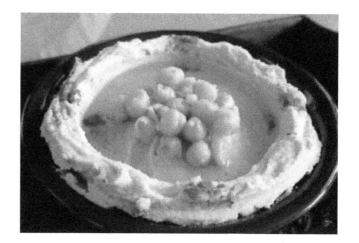

Nutrition:

Calories 129; Total Fat 7.4 g;

Saturated Fat 0.9 g; Cholesterol 0 mg;

Sodium 19521 mg; Total Carbs 12.2 g;

Fiber 3.3 g; Sugar 1.2 g; Protein 4.7 g

Preparation Time: 10 minutes

Cooking Time: 0 minutes

Servings: 12

Ingredients:

- 2 (15-ounce) cans chickpeas, rinsed and drained
- ½ cup tahini
- 1 garlic clove, chopped
- 2 tablespoons fresh lemon juice
- Sea salt, to taste
- Filtered water, as needed
- 1 tablespoon olive oil plus more for drizzling
- Pinch of cayenne pepper

Directions:

1. In a blender, add all the ingredients and pulse until smooth.
2. Transfer the hummus into a large bowl and drizzle with oil.
3. Sprinkle with cayenne pepper and serve immediately.

Smoothies, Teas, And Juices

160. Blueberry Smoothie

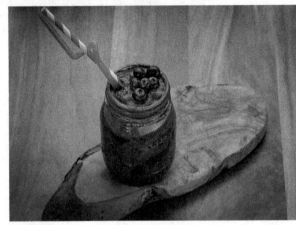

Preparation Time: 10 minutes

Cooking Time: 0 minutes

Servings: 2

Ingredients:

- 2 cups frozen blueberries
- 1 small banana
- 1½ cups unsweetened almond milk
- ¼ cup ice cubes

Directions:

1. Place all the ingredients in a high-speed blender and pulse until creamy.
2. Pour the smoothie into two glasses and serve immediately.

Nutrition: Calories 158 Total Fat 3.3 g Saturated Fat 0.3 g Cholesterol 0 mg Sodium 137 mg Total Carbs 34 g Fiber 5.6 g Sugar 20.6 g Protein 2.4 g

161. Raspberry and Tofu Smoothie

Preparation Time: 10 minutes

Cooking Time: 0 minutes

Servings: 2

Ingredients:

- 1½ cups fresh raspberries
- 6 ounces firm silken tofu, pressed and drained
- 4-5 drops liquid stevia
- 1 cup coconut cream
- ¼ cup ice, crushed

Directions:

1. Place all the ingredients in a high-speed blender and pulse until creamy.
2. Pour the smoothie into two glasses and serve immediately.

Nutrition: Calories 377 Total Fat 31.5 g Saturated Fat 25.7 g Cholesterol 0 mg Sodium 50 mg Total Carbs 19.7 g Fiber 8.7 g Sugar 9.2 g Protein 9.7 g

162. Beet and Strawberry Smoothie

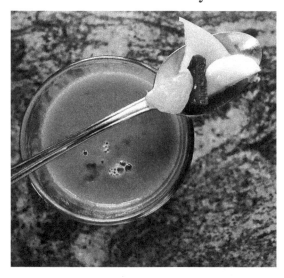

Preparation Time: 10 minutes

Cooking Time: 0 minutes

Servings: 2

Ingredients:

- 2 cups frozen strawberries, pitted and chopped
- 2/3 cup roasted and frozen beet, chopped
- 1 teaspoon fresh ginger, peeled and grated
- 1 teaspoon fresh turmeric, peeled and grated
- ½ cup fresh orange juice
- 1 cup unsweetened almond milk

Directions:

1. Place all the ingredients in a high-speed blender and pulse until creamy.
2. Pour the smoothie into two glasses and serve immediately.

Nutrition: Calories 258 Total Fat 1.5 g Saturated Fat 0.1 g Cholesterol 0 mg Sodium 134 mg Total Carbs 26.7g Fiber 4.9 g Sugar 18.7 g Protein 2.9 g

163. Kiwi Smoothie

Preparation Time: 10 minutes

Cooking Time: 0 minutes

Servings: 2

Ingredients:

- 4 kiwis
- 2 small bananas, peeled
- 1½ cups unsweetened almond milk
- 1-2 drops liquid stevia
- ¼ cup ice cubes

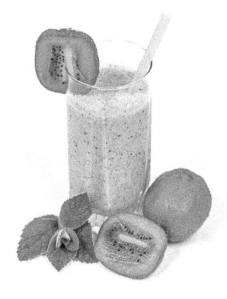

Directions:

1. Place all the ingredients in a high-speed blender and pulse until creamy.
2. Pour the smoothie into two glasses and serve immediately.

Nutrition: Calories 228 Total Fat 3.8 g Saturated Fat 0.4 g Cholesterol 0 mg Sodium 141 mg Total Carbs 50.7 g Fiber 8.4 g Sugar 28.1 g Protein 3.8 g

164. Pineapple and Carrot Smoothie

Preparation Time: 10 minutes

Cooking Time: 0 minutes

Servings: 2

Ingredients:

- 1 cup frozen pineapple
- 1 large ripe banana, peeled and sliced
- ½ tablespoon fresh ginger, peeled and chopped
- ¼ teaspoon ground turmeric
- 1 cup unsweetened almond milk
- ½ cup fresh carrot juice
- 1 tablespoon fresh lemon juice

Directions:

1. Place all the ingredients in a high-speed blender and pulse until creamy.
2. Pour the smoothie into two glasses and serve immediately.

Nutrition: Calories 132 Total Fat 2.2 g Saturated Fat 0.3 g Cholesterol 0 mg Sodium 113 mg Total Carbs 629.3 g Fiber 4.1 g Sugar 16.9 g Protein 2 g

165. Oats and Orange Smoothie

Preparation Time: 10 minutes

Cooking Time: 0 minutes

Servings: 4

Ingredients:

- 2/3 cup rolled oats
- 2 oranges, peeled, seeded, and sectioned
- 2 large bananas, peeled and sliced
- 2 cups unsweetened almond milk
- 1 cup ice cubes, crushed

Directions:

1. Place all the ingredients in a high-speed blender and pulse until creamy.
2. Pour the smoothie into four glasses and serve immediately.

Nutrition: Calories 175; Total Fat 3 g Saturated Fat 0.4 g Cholesterol 0 mg Sodium 93 mg Total Carbs 36.6 g Fiber 5.9 g Sugar 17.1 g Protein 3.9 g

166. Pumpkin Smoothie

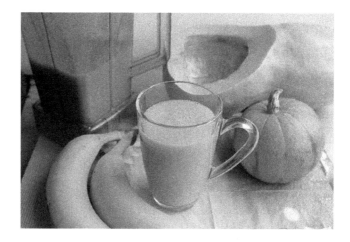

Preparation Time: 10 minutes

Cooking Time: 0 minutes

Servings: 2

Ingredients:

- 1 cup homemade pumpkin puree
- 1 medium banana, peeled and sliced
- 1 tablespoon maple syrup
- 1 teaspoon ground flaxseeds
- ½ teaspoon ground cinnamon
- ¼ teaspoon ground ginger
- 1½ cups unsweetened almond milk
- ¼ cup ice cubes

Directions:

1. Place all the ingredients in a high-speed blender and pulse until creamy.
2. Pour the smoothie into two glasses and serve immediately.

Nutrition: Calories 159 Total Fat 3.6 g Saturated Fat 0.5 g Cholesterol 0 mg Sodium 143 mg Total Carbs 32.6 g Fiber 6.5 g Sugar 17.3 g Protein 3 g

167. Red Veggie and Fruit Smoothie

Preparation Time: 10 minutes

Cooking Time: 0 minutes

Servings: 2

Ingredients:

- ½ cup fresh raspberries
- ½ cup fresh strawberries
- ½ red bell pepper, seeded and chopped
- ½ cup red cabbage, chopped
- 1 small tomato
- 1 cup water
- ½ cup ice cubes

Directions:

1. Place all the ingredients in a high-speed blender and pulse until creamy.
2. Pour the smoothie into two glasses and serve immediately.

Nutrition: Calories 39 Cholesterol 0 mg Saturated Fat 0 g Sodium 10 mg Total Carbs 8.9 g Fiber 3.5 g Sugar 4.8 g Protein 1.3 g Total Fat 0.4 g

168. Kale Smoothie

Preparation Time: 10 minutes

Cooking Time: 0 minutes

Servings: 2

Ingredients:

- 3 stalks fresh kale, trimmed and chopped
- 1-2 celery stalks, chopped
- ½ avocado, peeled, pitted, and chopped
- ½-inch piece ginger root, chopped
- ½-inch piece turmeric root, chopped
- 2 cups coconut milk

Directions:

1. Place all the ingredients in a high-speed blender and pulse until creamy.
2. Pour the smoothie into two glasses and serve immediately.

Nutrition: Calories 248 Total Fat 21.8 g Saturated Fat 12 g Cholesterol 0 mg Sodium 59 mg Total Carbs 11.3 g Fiber 4.2 g Sugar 0.5 g Protein 3.5 g

169. Green Tofu Smoothie

Preparation Time: 10 minutes

Cooking Time: 0 minutes

Servings: 2

Ingredients:

- 1½ cups cucumber, peeled and chopped roughly
- 3 cups fresh baby spinach
- 2 cups frozen broccoli
- ½ cup silken tofu, drained and pressed
- 1 tablespoon fresh lime juice
- 4-5 drops liquid stevia

- 1 cup unsweetened almond milk
- ½ cup ice, crushed

Directions:

1. Place all the ingredients in a high-speed blender and pulse until creamy.
2. Pour the smoothie into two glasses and serve immediately.

Nutrition: Calories 118 Total Fat 15 g Saturated Fat 0.8 g Cholesterol 0 mg Sodium 165 mg Total Carbs 12.6 g Fiber 4.8 g Sugar 3.4 g Protein 10 g

170. Grape and Swiss Chard Smoothie

Preparation Time: 10 minutes

Cooking Time: 0 minutes

Servings: 2

Ingredients:

- 2 cups seedless green grapes
- 2 cups fresh Swiss chard, trimmed and chopped
- 2 tablespoons maple syrup
- 1 teaspoon fresh lemon juice
- 1½ cups water
- 4 ice cubes

Directions:

1. Place all the ingredients in a high-speed blender and pulse until creamy.
2. Pour the smoothie into two glasses and serve immediately.

Nutrition: Calories 176 Total Fat 0.2 g Saturated Fat 0 g Cholesterol 0 mg Sodium 83 mg Total Carbs 44.9 g Fiber 1.7 g Sugar 37.9 g Protein 0.7 g

171. Matcha Smoothie

Preparation Time: 10 minutes

Cooking Time: 0 minutes

Servings: 2

Ingredients:

- 2 tablespoons chia seeds
- 2 teaspoons Matcha green tea powder
- ½ teaspoon fresh lemon juice
- ½ teaspoon xanthan gum

- 8-10 drops liquid stevia
- 4 tablespoons coconut cream
- 1½ cups unsweetened almond milk
- ¼ cup ice cubes

Directions:

1. Place all the ingredients in a high-speed blender and pulse until creamy.
2. Pour the smoothie into two glasses and serve immediately.

Nutrition: Calories 132 Total Fat 12.3 g Saturated Fat 6.8 g Cholesterol 0 mg Sodium 15 mg Total Carbs 7 g Fiber 4.8 g Sugar 1 g Protein 3 g

172. Banana Smoothie

Preparation Time: 10 minutes

Cooking Time: 0 minutes

Servings: 2

Ingredients:

- 2 cups chilled unsweetened almond milk
- 1 large frozen banana, peeled and sliced
- 1 tablespoon almonds, chopped
- 1 teaspoon organic vanilla extract

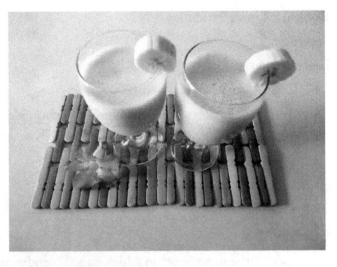

Directions:

1. Place all the ingredients in a high-speed blender and pulse until creamy.
2. Pour the smoothie into two glasses and serve immediately.

Nutrition:

Calories 124, Total Fat 5.2 g, Saturated Fat 0.5 g, Cholesterol 0 mg

Sodium 181 mg, Total Carbs 18.4 g

Fiber 3.1 g, Sugar 8.7 g, Protein 2.4 g

173. Strawberry Smoothie

Nutrition:

Calories 131; Total Fat 3.7 g

Saturated Fat 0.4 g; Cholesterol 0 mg

Sodium 181 mg; Total Carbs 25.3 g

Fiber 4.8 g; Sugar 14 g; Protein 1.6 g

Preparation Time: 10 minutes

Cooking Time: 0 minutes

Servings: 2

Ingredients:

- 2 cups chilled unsweetened almond milk
- 1½ cups frozen strawberries
- 1 banana, peeled and sliced
- ¼ teaspoon organic vanilla extract

Directions:

1. Add all the ingredients in a high-speed blender and pulse until smooth.
2. Pour the smoothie into two glasses and serve immediately.

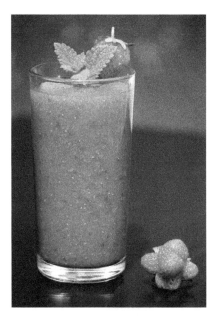

174. Raspberry and Tofu Smoothie

Preparation Time: 15 minutes

Cooking Time: 0 minutes

Servings: 2

Ingredients:

- 1½ cups fresh raspberries
- 6 ounces firm silken tofu, drained
- 1/8 teaspoon coconut extract
- 1 teaspoon powdered stevia
- 1½ cups unsweetened almond milk
- ¼ cup ice cubes, crushed

Directions:

1. Add all the ingredients in a high-speed blender and pulse until smooth.
2. Pour the smoothie into two glasses and serve immediately.

Nutrition:

Calories 131, Total Fat 5.5 g, Saturated Fat 0.6 g

Cholesterol 0 mg, Sodium 167 mg, Total Carbs 14.6 g

Fiber 6.8 g, Sugar 5.2 g, Protein 7.7 g

175. Mango Smoothie

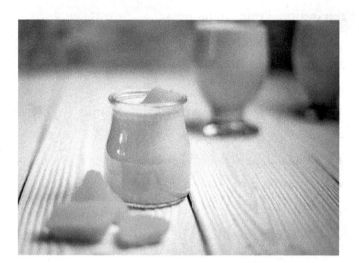

Preparation Time: 10 minutes

Cooking Time: 0 minutes

Servings: 2

Ingredients:

- 2 cups frozen mango, peeled, pitted and chopped
- ¼ cup almond butter
- Pinch of ground turmeric
- 2 tablespoons fresh lemon juice
- 1¼ cups unsweetened almond milk
- ¼ cup ice cubes

Directions:

1. Add all the ingredients in a high-speed blender and pulse until smooth.
2. Pour the smoothie into two glasses and serve immediately.

Nutrition: Calories 140 Total Fat 4.1 g Saturated Fat 0.6 g Cholesterol 0 mg Sodium 118 mg Total Carbs 26.8 g Fiber 3.6 g Sugar 23 g Protein 2.5 g

176. Pineapple Smoothie

Preparation Time: 10 minutes

Cooking Time: 0 minutes

Servings: 2

Ingredients:

- 2 cups pineapple, chopped
- ½ teaspoon fresh ginger, peeled and chopped
- ½ teaspoon ground turmeric
- 1 teaspoon natural immune support supplement
- 1 teaspoon chia seeds
- 1½ cups cold green tea
- ½ cup ice, crushed

Directions:

1. Add all the ingredients in a high-speed blender and pulse until smooth.
2. Pour the smoothie into two glasses and serve immediately.

Nutrition: Calories 152 Total Fat 1 g Saturated Fat 0 g Cholesterol 0 mg

Sodium 9 mg Total Carbs 30 g Fiber 3.5 g Sugar 29.8 g Protein 1.5 g

177. Kale and Pineapple Smoothie

Preparation Time: 15 minutes

Cooking Time: 0 minutes

Servings: 2

Ingredients:

- 1½ cups fresh kale, trimmed and chopped
- 1 frozen banana, peeled and chopped
- ½ cup fresh pineapple chunks
- 1 cup unsweetened coconut milk
- ½ cup fresh orange juice
- ½ cup ice

Directions:

1. Add all the ingredients in a high-speed blender and pulse until smooth.
2. Pour the smoothie into two glasses and serve immediately.

Nutrition: Calories 148 Total Fat 2.4 g Saturated Fat 2.1 g

Cholesterol 0 mg Sodium 23 mg Total Carbs 31.6 g

Fiber 3.5 g Sugar 16.5 g Protein 2.8 g

178. Green Veggies Smoothie

Preparation Time: 15 minutes

Cooking Time: 0 minutes

Servings: 2

Ingredients:

- 1 medium avocado, peeled, pitted, and chopped
- 1 large cucumber, peeled and chopped
- 2 fresh tomatoes, chopped
- 1 small green bell pepper, seeded and chopped
- 1 cup fresh spinach, torn
- 2 tablespoons fresh lime juice
- 2 tablespoons homemade vegetable broth
- 1 cup alkaline water

Directions:

1. Add all the ingredients in a high-speed blender and pulse until smooth.

2. Pour the smoothie into glasses and serve immediately.

Nutrition: Calories 275 Total Fat 20.3 g Saturated Fat 4.2 g Cholesterol 0 mg Sodium 76 mg Total Carbs 24.1 g Fiber 10.1 g Sugar 9.3 g Protein 5.3 g

179. Avocado and Spinach Smoothie

Preparation Time: 10 minutes

Cooking Time: 0 minutes

Servings: 2

Ingredients:

- 2 cups fresh baby spinach
- ½ avocado, peeled, pitted, and chopped
- 4-6 drops liquid stevia
- ½ teaspoon ground cinnamon
- 1 tablespoon hemp seeds
- 2 cups chilled alkaline water

Directions:

1. Add all the ingredients in a high-speed blender and pulse until smooth.

2. Pour the smoothie into two glasses and serve immediately.

Nutrition: Calories 132 Total Fat 11.7 g Saturated Fat 2.2 g Cholesterol 0 mg Sodium 27 mg Total Carbs 6.1 g Fiber 4.5 g Sugar 0.4 g Protein 3.1 g

180. Cucumber Smoothie

Preparation Time: 15 minutes

Cooking Time: 0 minutes

Servings: 2

Ingredients:

- 1 small cucumber, peeled and chopped
- 2 cups mixed fresh greens (spinach, kale, beet greens), trimmed and chopped
- ½ cup lettuce, torn
- ¼ cup fresh parsley leaves
- ¼ cup fresh mint leaves
- 2-3 drops liquid stevia

- 1 teaspoon fresh lemon juice
- 1½ cups filtered water
- ¼ cup ice cubes

Directions:

1. Add all the ingredients in a high-speed blender and pulse until smooth.
2. Pour the smoothie into two glasses and serve immediately.

Nutrition: Calories 50 Total Fat 0.5 g Saturated Fat 0.2 g Cholesterol 0 mg Sodium 34 mg Total Carbs 11.3 g Fiber 3.6 g Sugar 3.2 g Protein 2.5 g

181. Apple Ginger Smoothie

Preparation Time: 10 minutes

Cooking Time: 0 minutes

Servings: 1

Ingredients:

- 1 Apple, peeled and diced
- ¾ cup (6 oz) coconut yogurt
- ½ teaspoon ginger, freshly grated

Directions:

1. Add all the ingredients to a blender.
2. Blend well until smooth.
3. Refrigerate for 2 to 3 hours.
4. Serve.

Nutrition: Calories 144; Total Fat 0.4 g; Saturated Fat 5 g; Cholesterol 51 mg; Sodium 86 mg; Total Carbs 8 g; Fiber 2.3 g; Sugar 2.2 g; Protein 5.6 g.

182. Green Tea Blueberry Smoothie

Nutrition: Calories 144, Total Fat 0.4 g,

Saturated Fat 5 g, Cholesterol 51 mg,

Sodium 86 mg, Total Carbs 8 g,

Fiber 2.3 g Sugar 2.2 g Protein 5.6 g

Preparation Time: 10 minutes

Cooking Time: 5 minutes

Servings: 1

Ingredients:

- 3 tablespoons alkaline water
- 1 green tea bag
- 1½ cup fresh blueberries
- 1 pear, peeled, cored and diced
- ¾ cup almond milk

Directions:

1. Boil 3 tablespoons water in a small pot and transfer it to a cup.
2. Dip the tea bag in the cup and let it sit for 4 to 5 mins.
3. Discard tea bag and
4. Transfer the green tea to a blender
5. Add all the remaining the ingredients to the blender.
6. Blend well until smooth.
7. Serve with fresh blueberries.

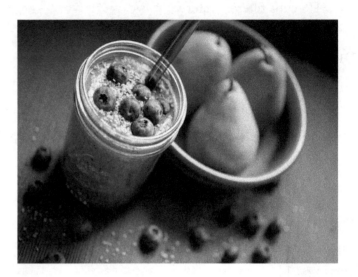

183. Apple Almond Smoothie

Preparation Time: 10 minutes

Cooking Time: 0 minutes

Servings: 1

Ingredients:

- 1 cup apple cider
- 1/2 cup coconut yogurt
- 4 tablespoons almonds, crushed
- 1/4 teaspoon cinnamon
- 1/4 teaspoon nutmeg
- 1 cup ice cubes

Directions:

1. Add all the ingredients to a blender.
2. Blend well until smooth.
3. Serve.

Nutrition: Calories 144 Total Fat 0.4 g Saturated Fat 5 g;

Cholesterol 51 mg Sodium 86 mg Total Carbs 8 g Fiber 2.3 g Sugar 2.2 g Protein 5.6 g

184. Cranberry Smoothie

Preparation Time: 10 minutes

Cooking Time: 0 minutes

Servings: 1

Ingredients:

- 1 cup cranberries
- ¾ cup almond milk
- ¼ cup raspberries
- 2 teaspoon fresh ginger, finely grated
- 2 teaspoons fresh lemon juice

Directions:

1. Add all the ingredients to a blender.
2. Blend well until smooth.
3. Serve with fresh berries on top.

Nutrition: Calories 144 Total Fat 0.4 g Saturated Fat 5 g Cholesterol 51 mg Sodium 86 mg Total Carbs 8 g Fiber 2.3 g Sugar 2.2 g Protein 5.6 g

185. Cinnamon Berry Smoothie

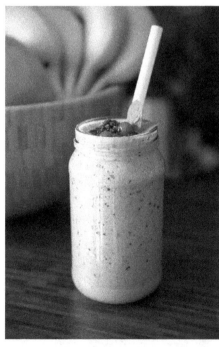

Preparation Time: 10 minutes

Cooking Time: 0 minutes

Servings: 01

Ingredients:

- 1 cup frozen strawberries
- 1 cup apple, peeled and diced
- 2 teaspoon fresh ginger
- 3 tablespoons hemp seeds
- 1 cup water
- ½ lime juiced
- ¼ teaspoon cinnamon powder
- 1/8 teaspoon vanilla extract

Directions:

1. Add all the ingredients to a blender.

2. Blend well until smooth.

3. Serve with fresh fruits

Nutrition:

Calories 144, Total Fat 0.4 g, Saturated Fat 5 g,

Cholesterol 51 mg, Sodium 86 mg, Total Carbs 8 g,

Fiber 2.3 g, Sugar 2.2 g, Protein 5.6 g

186. Detox Berries smoothie

Preparation Time: 10 minutes

Cooking Time: 0 minutes

Servings: 1

Ingredients:

- 3 peaches, cored and peeled
- 5 blueberries
- 5 raspberries
- 1 cup alkaline water

Directions:

1. Add all the ingredients to a blender.

2. Blend well until smooth.

3. Serve with fresh kiwi wedges.

Nutrition:

Calories 144, Total Fat 0.4 g,

Saturated Fat 5 g, Cholesterol 51 mg,

Sodium 86 mg, Total Carbs 8 g,

Fiber 2.3 g, Sugar 2.2 g, Protein 5.6 g

187. Pink Smoothie

Preparation Time: 10 minutes

Cooking Time: 0 minutes

Servings: 1

Ingredients:

- 1 peach, cored and peeled

- 6 ripe strawberries
- 1 cup almond milk

Directions:

1. Add all the ingredients to a blender.

2. Blend well until smooth.

3. Serve with your favorite berries

Nutrition:

Calories 144, Total Fat 0.4 g,

Saturated Fat 5 g, Cholesterol 51 mg,

Sodium 86 mg, Total Carbs 8 g,

Fiber 2.3 g, Sugar 2.2 g, Protein 5.6 g

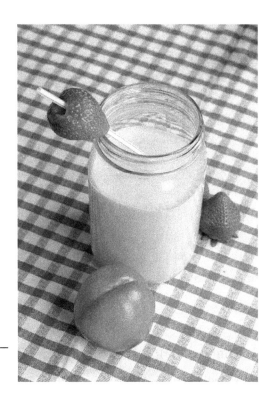

188. Green Apple Smoothie

Preparation Time: 10 minutes

Cooking Time: 0 minutes

Servings: 1

Ingredients:

- 1 peach, peeled and cored
- 1 green apple, peeled and cored
- 1 cup alkaline water

Directions:

1. Add all the ingredients to a blender.

2. Blend well until smooth.

3. Serve with apple slices.

Nutrition:

Calories 144, Total Fat 0.4 g,

Saturated Fat 5 g, Cholesterol 51 mg,

Sodium 86 mg, Total Carbs 8 g,

Fiber 2.3 g, Sugar 2.2 g, Protein 5.6 g

189. Avocado Smoothie

Preparation Time: 10 minutes

Cooking Time: 0 minutes

Servings: 1

Ingredients:

- 1 carrot, grated
- 1 avocado, cored and peeled
- ½ pear, cored
- ½ cup blackberries
- 1 ½ cups unsweetened almond milk

Directions:

1. Add all the ingredients to a blender.
2. Blend well until smooth.
3. Serve with blackberries on top.

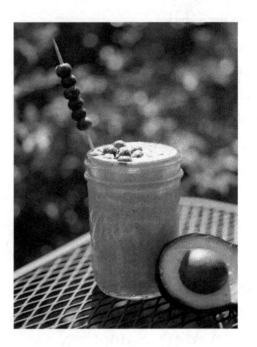

Nutrition: Calories 144 Total Fat 0.4 g Saturated Fat 5 g Cholesterol 51 mg Sodium 86 mg Total Carbs 8 g Fiber 2.3 g Sugar 2.2 g Protein 5.6 g

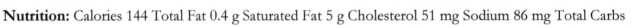

190. Green Smoothie

Preparation Time: 10 minutes

Cooking Time: 0 minutes

Servings: 1

Ingredients:

- 1 cup alkaline water
- 3/4 cup raw coconut water
- 1/2 teaspoon probiotic powder
- 2 cups firmly packed baby spinach
- 1 cup raw young Thai coconut meat
- 1 avocado, peeled and pitted
- 1/2 cucumber, chopped-chopped
- 1 teaspoon lime zest, finely grated
- 2 limes
- Stevia, to taste
- Pinch of Celtic sea salt

- 2 cups ice cubes

Directions:

1. Add all the ingredients to a blender.
2. Blend well until smooth.
3. Serve with an avocado slice on top.

Nutrition:

Calories 144, Total Fat 0.4 g,

Saturated Fat 5 g, Cholesterol 51 mg,

Sodium 86 mg, Total Carbs 8 g,

Fiber 2.3 g, Sugar 2.2 g, Protein 5.6 g

191. Spiced Banana Smoothie

Preparation Time: 5 minutes

Cooking Time: 0 minutes

Servings: 2

Ingredients:

- 2 medium frozen bananas, peeled and sliced
- 1 tsp organic vanilla extract
- ¼ tsp ground cinnamon
- Pinch of ground nutmeg
- Pinch of ground cloves
- 1½ cups unsweetened almond milk

Directions:

1. Place all the ingredients in a high-speed blender and pulse until creamy.
2. Pour the smoothie into two glasses and serve immediately.

Nutrition:

Calories 143; Total Fat 2.1 g;

Saturated Fat 0.4 g; Sodium 137 mg;

Fiber 4 g; Sugar 14.8 g; Protein 2.1 g;

Cholesterol 0 mg; Total Carbs 29.1 g

192. Blueberry Smoothie

Preparation Time: 5 minutes.

Cooking Time: 0 minutes

Servings: 2

Ingredients:

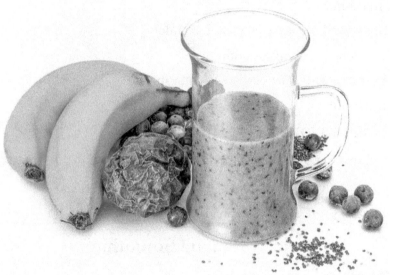

- 2 cups frozen blueberries
- 1½ cups unsweetened almond milk
- 1 small banana, peeled and sliced
- ¼ cup ice cubes

Directions:

1. Place all the ingredients in a high-speed blender and pulse until creamy.
2. Serve immediately after pouring the smoothie into two glasses.

Nutrition: Calories 158; Saturated Fat 0.3 g; Sodium 137 mg; Total Carbs 34 g; Fiber 5.6 g; Sugar 20 g; Protein 2.2 g; Total Fat 3.3 g; Cholesterol 0 mg

193. Raspberry and Tofu Smoothie

Preparation Time: 10 minutes.

Cooking Time: 0 minutes

Servings: 2

Ingredients:

- 8 oz firm silken tofu, pressed and drained
- 1 cup frozen raspberries
- ¼ tsp coconut extract
- 4-6 drops liquid stevia
- 1 cup coconut cream
- ½ cup ice cubes, crushed

Directions:

1. Place all the ingredients in a high-speed blender and pulse until creamy.
2. Pour the smoothie into two glasses and serve immediately.

Nutrition: Calories 328; Saturated Fat 9.7 g; Sodium 32 mg; Total Carbs 39.4 g;

Fiber 6.5 g; Sugar 28 g; Protein 11.4g; Total Fat 15.4 g; Cholesterol 0 mg

194. Papaya Smoothie

Preparation Time: 10 minutes.

Cooking Time: 0 minutes

Servings: 2

Ingredients:

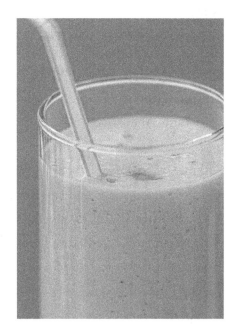

- 1 large banana, peeled and sliced
- ½ medium papaya, peeled and chopped roughly
- 1½ cups unsweetened almond milk
- 2 tbsp agave syrup
- 1 tbsp fresh lime juice
- ¼ tsp ground turmeric
- ½ cup ice cubes, crushed

Directions:

1. Place all the ingredients in a high-speed blender and pulse until creamy.

2. Pour the smoothie into two glasses and serve immediately.

Nutrition: Calories 190; Total Fat 3.1 g; Saturated Fat 0.4 g; Sodium 157 mg; Total Carbs 42.6 g; Sugar 14.5 g; Protein 1.9 g; Cholesterol 0 mg; Fiber 3.9 g

195. Peach Smoothie

Preparation Time: 10 minutes.

Cooking Time: 0 minutes

Servings: 2

Ingredients:

- 1 large peach, peeled, pitted, and chopped
- 1 medium frozen banana, peeled and sliced
- 2 oz Aloe Vera
- ½ tsp fresh ginger, peeled and chopped
- 2 tbsp flax seeds
- ½ tsp organic vanilla extract
- 1¾ cups unsweetened almond milk

Directions:

1. Add all the ingredients in a high-speed blender and pulse until smooth.

2. Pour the smoothie into two glasses and serve immediately.

Nutrition: Calories 162; Saturated Fat 0.6g; Sodium 160mg; Total Carbs 25.7g; Fiber 5.5 g; Sugar 14.5 g; Protein 3.6 g; Cholesterol 0mg; Total Fat 5.7g

196. Strawberry and Beet Smoothie

Preparation Time: 10 minutes.

Cooking Time: 0 minutes

Servings: 2

Ingredients:

- 2 cups frozen strawberries, pitted and chopped
- 2/3 cup frozen beets, chopped
- 1 tsp fresh ginger, peeled and grated
- 1 tsp fresh turmeric, peeled and grated
- ½ cup fresh orange juice
- 1 cup unsweetened almond milk

Directions:

1. Add all the ingredients in a high-speed blender and pulse until smooth.
2. Pour the smoothie into two glasses and serve immediately.

Nutrition: Calories 130; Saturated Fat 0.2 g; Sodium 135 mg; Total Carbs 27.5 g; Fiber 5.1 g; Sugar 18.7 g; Protein 2 g; Cholesterol 0 mg; Total Fat 2.1 g

197. Grape and Swiss Chard Smoothie

Preparation Time: 10 minutes.

Cooking Time: 0 minutes

Servings: 2

Ingredients:

- 2 cups seedless green grapes
- 2 cups fresh Swiss chard, trimmed and chopped
- 2 tbsp agave nectar
- 1 tsp fresh lemon juice
- 1½ cups alkaline water
- ¼ cup ice cubes, crushed

Directions:

1. Add all the ingredients in a high-speed blender and pulse until smooth.

2. Pour the smoothie into two glasses and serve immediately.

Nutrition: Calories 128; Saturated Fat 0 g; Sodium 78 mg; Total Carbs 33.4 g; Fiber 2.6 g; Sugar 30.5 g; Protein 1.7g; Cholesterol 0 mg; Total Fat 1.1 g

198. Green Veggie Smoothie 2

Preparation Time: 10 minutes.

Cooking Time: 0 minutes

Servings: 2

Ingredients:

- ½ small cucumber, peeled and chopped roughly
- 1 cup fresh dandelion greens, chopped
- 1 celery stalk, chopped
- ¼ tsp fresh ginger, chopped
- 8-10 drops liquid stevia
- ½ tbsp fresh lime juice
- 1½ cups alkaline water
- ¼ cup ice cubes, crushed

Directions:

1. Add all the ingredients in a high-speed blender and pulse until smooth.
2. Pour the smoothie into two glasses and serve immediately.

Nutrition: Calories 26; Saturated Fat 0.1 g; Sodium 30 mg; Total Carbs 5.7 g; Fiber 1.5 g; Sugar 1.6 g; Protein 1.3 g; Cholesterol 0 mg; Total Fat 0.3 g

199. Pepper Mint Tea Surprise

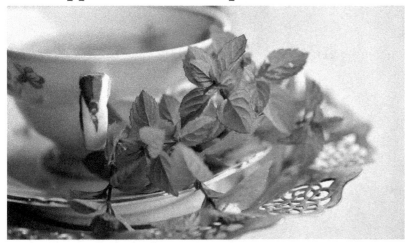

Preparation Time: 4 minutes

Cooking Time: 15 minutes

Servings: 2

Ingredients:

- 1 tablespoon peppermint leaves
- 1 tablespoon regular mint
- 1 tablespoon basil leaves
- A few dates, pitted
- 2 cups alkaline water

Directions:

1. Boil the water.

2. Place the tea ingredients and the dates in a tea pot or teacup.

3. Pour over some boiling water and cover.

4. Leave covered for 15 minutes.

5. Strain all the ingredients and serve in a nice teacup.

6. Feel free to throw in the dates back (yummy!). You can also re-use them to make a smoothie, using some of the recipes in this book that call for dates.

Nutrition: Calories 22; Saturated Fat 0.3 g; Sodium 20 mg; Total Carbs 4.7 g; Fiber 1.6 g; Sugar 1.0 g; Protein 3.3 g

200. Chamomile Tea with Parsley

Preparation Time: 3 minutes

Cooking Time: 15 minutes

Servings: 2

Ingredients:

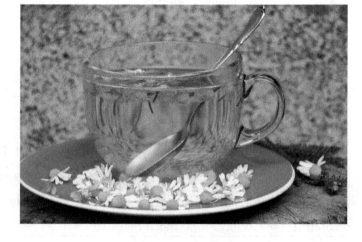

- 2 tablespoons chamomile flowers
- 2 tablespoons parsley
- 2 cups alkaline water
- A few mint leaves to garnish

Directions:

1. Boil the water.

2. Place the tea ingredients in a tea pot or teacup.

3. Pour over the boiling water and cover.

4. Leave covered for 15 minutes.

5. Strain all the ingredients and serve in a nice teacup.

6. Garnish with some mint leaves.

7. Enjoy!

Nutrition:

Calories 12; Saturated Fat 0.2 g; Sodium 11mg; Total Carbs 4.7 g; Fiber 1.3 g; Sugar 2.0 g; Protein 2 g

201. Lavender Mint Tea

Preparation Time: 5 minutes

Cooking Time: 5 minutes

Servings: 2-4

Ingredients:

- 2 tablespoons lavender flowers
- 2 tablespoons mint leaves
- 4 cups alkaline water

Directions:

1. Clean the lavender flowers thoroughly under running water.
2. Chop it roughly and place it in a large saucepan.
3. Clean and roughly chop the mint leaves and add to the saucepan.
4. Add the water to the pan and allow it to come to a boil.
5. Once it starts to boil, lower the heat and simmer for 5 minutes.
6. Strain and pour into a mug.
7. Serve and enjoy!

Nutrition:

Calories 18; Saturated Fat 02 g; Sodium 13 mg; Total Carbs 7 g; Fiber 6 g; Sugar 0 g; Protein 1.3 g

202. Almond Milk and Rosemary Tea

Preparation Time: 2 minutes

Cooking Time: 5 minutes

Servings: 2

Ingredients:

- 2 cups almond milk
- 4 tablespoons rosemary herb
- A few bananas slice
- A few apples slice
- 1 tablespoon coconut oil

Directions:

1. Heat the almond milk in a saucepan.
2. Place the rest of the ingredients in a tea pot or a teacup.
3. Pour over the boiling milk.
4. Cover for 15 minutes.
5. Strain and pour into a teacup.
6. Enjoy!

Nutrition:

Calories 25; Saturated Fat 3 g; Sodium 21 mg; Total Carbs 1.7 g; Fiber 2 g; Sugar 0 .4g; Protein 1.3 g

203. Cucumber Infused Lemon Iced Tea

Preparation Time: 8 minutes,

Cooking Time: 10 minutes

Servings: 2-3

Ingredients:

- 2 cups cucumber
- 3 cups alkaline water
- 1 cup lemon juice
- Stevia to sweeten (optional)
- Ice cubes
- Mint leaves

Directions:

1. Boil one cup of water.
2. Clean the cucumber thoroughly and remove the pith from both ends.
3. Cut it into thin circles or little pieces.
4. Place it in a bowl and add stevia (optional).
5. Pour the hot water on top and allow it to rest for 10 minutes.
6. Meanwhile, mix the two cups of water and the lemon juice and place it in the fridge.
7. Crush the ice in a coffee grinder or blender.
8. Strain the cucumber water and add the ice cubes.
9. Add in the cold lemon juice. Sprinkle some roughly chopped mint leaves on top and serve.

Nutrition:

Calories 30; Saturated Fat 0.8 g; Sodium 25 mg; Total Carbs 4.2 g; Fiber 1.4 g; Sugar 1.6 g; Protein 3.1 g

Buddha Bowl Recipes

204. Strawberry and Chia Seed Overnight Oats Parfait

Preparation Time: 10 minutes

Cooking Time: 0 minutes

Servings: 2

Ingredients:

FOR STRAWBERRY MIXTURE:

- 1 cup diced strawberries
- 1 teaspoon chia seeds
- 1 to 2 teaspoons brown rice syrup

FOR OAT MIXTURE:

- 1 cup quick rolled oats
- 1 cup coconut milk (boxed)
- 1 tablespoon brown rice syrup
- 1/8 tablespoon vanilla bean powder

Directions:

Strawberry mixture:

1. In a small bowl, stir together the strawberries, chia seeds, and brown rice syrup until well combined.

Oat mixture:

2. In a small bowl, stir together the oats, coconut milk, brown rice syrup, and vanilla bean powder until well combined.
3. Place half the oat mixture in the bottom of 1 large glass mason jar or 2 small jars, and layer half of the strawberry mixture over the oat mixture. Repeat with the remaining oat and strawberry mixtures.
4. Cover the mason jar and refrigerate overnight.
5. Uncover and enjoy.

Nutrition:

Calories: 245 kcal

Fat: 6g

Carbs: 12g

Protein: 8g

205. Carrot and Hemp Seed Muffins

Preparation Time: 5 minutes

Cooking Time: 25 minutes

Servings: 12

Ingredients:

- 3 tablespoons water
- 1 tablespoon ground flaxseed
- 2 cups oat flour
- 1 cup almond milk (boxed)
- ½ cup unrefined whole cane sugar
- 1 carrot, shredded
- 6 tablespoons cashew butter
- 2 tablespoons hemp seeds
- 1 tablespoon chopped Lacinato kale
- 1 tablespoon baking powder
- 1/8 teaspoon vanilla bean powder
- Pinch sea salt

Directions:

1. Preheat the oven to 350°F.
2. To prepare a flax egg, in a small bowl, whisk together the water and flaxseed.
3. Transfer the flax egg to a medium bowl, and add the oat flour, almond milk, sugar, carrot, cashew butter, hemp seeds, kale, baking powder, vanilla bean powder, and salt, stirring until well combined.
4. Divide the mixture evenly among 12 muffin cups, bake for 20 to 25 minutes, and enjoy right away.

Nutrition:

Calories: 334 kcal

Fat: 5.6g

Carbs: 19.5g

Protein: 25.5g

206. Raspberry-Avocado Smoothie Bowl

Preparation Time: 5 minutes

Cooking Time: 0 minutes

Servings: 2

Ingredients:

- 1½ cups coconut milk (boxed)
- 1 cup raspberries, plus more (optional) for topping
- 1 avocado, roughly chopped
- 3 tablespoons unrefined whole cane sugar
- 1 teaspoon chia seeds
- 1 teaspoon unsweetened shredded coconut
- Mixed berries, for topping (optional)

Directions:

1. In a blender, blend the coconut milk, raspberries, avocado, and 2 tablespoons of sugar until smooth and creamy.

2. Pour the mixture into 2 serving bowls, sprinkle the extra raspberries (if using), the remaining 1 tablespoon of the sugar, chia seeds, shredded coconut, and mixed berries (if using) over the top, and enjoy.

Nutrition:

Calories: 145 kcal

Fat: 3.5g

Carbs: 5.7g

Protein: 6.7g

207. Sweet Potato and Kale Breakfast Hash

Preparation Time: 10 minutes

Cooking Time: 15 minutes

Servings: 2

Ingredients:

- 1 teaspoon avocado oil
- 2 cups peeled and cubed sweet potatoes
- ½ cup chopped kale
- ½ cup diced onion
- ½ teaspoon sea salt
- ½ teaspoon freshly ground black pepper
- ½ avocado, cubed (optional)
- 1 to 2 teaspoons sesame seeds or hemp seeds (optional)

Directions:

1. In a large skillet over medium heat, heat the avocado oil. Add the sweet potatoes, kale, onion, salt, and pepper, and sauté for 10 to 15 minutes, or until the sweet potatoes are soft. Remove from the heat.

2. Gently stir in the avocado and sesame seeds (if using), transfer to 1 large or 2 small plates, and enjoy.

Nutrition:

Calories: 176 kcal

Fat: 3.3g

Carbs: 14.8g

Protein: 17.0g

208. Avocados with Kale and Almond Stuffing

Preparation Time: 5 minutes

Cooking Time: 0 minutes

Servings: 2

Ingredients:

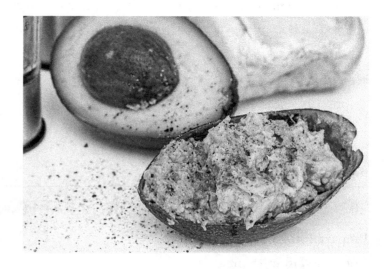

- ½ cup almonds
- ½ cup chopped Lacinato kale
- 1 garlic clove
- ½ jalapeño
- 2 tablespoons nutritional yeast
- 1 tablespoon avocado oil
- 1 tablespoon apple cider vinegar
- 1 tablespoon freshly squeezed lemon juice
- ¼ teaspoon sea salt
- 1 avocado, halved and pitted

Directions:

1. In a food processor, pulse the almonds, kale, garlic, jalapeño, nutritional yeast, avocado oil, apple cider vinegar, lemon juice, and sea salt until everything is well combined, the almonds are in small pieces, and it has a chunky texture, taking care not to over process.

2. Add half of the stuffing mixture to the center of each avocado half, and enjoy.

Nutrition:

Calories: 265 kcal

Fat: 1.1g

Carbs: 15.1g

Protein: 19.4g

209. Mixed Berry–Chia Seed Pudding

Preparation Time: 5 minutes

Cooking Time: 0 minutes

Servings: 1

Ingredients:

- 1 cup coconut milk (boxed)
- ½ cup mixed berries (raspberries, blackberries, blueberries), plus more (optional) for topping
- 2 tablespoons chia seeds
- 1 to 2 tablespoons unrefined whole cane sugar

Directions:

1. In a mason jar, combine the coconut milk, berries, chia seeds, and sugar, adjusting the sugar to your preference.
2. Seal the jar tightly and shake vigorously until well mixed.
3. Refrigerate for about 1 hour, or until the pudding thickens to your preference.
4. Stir, top with the extra mixed berries and enjoy.

Nutrition:

Calories: 316 kcal

Fat: 4.4g

Carbs: 10.6g

Protein: 16.4g

210. Pineapple and Coconut Oatmeal Bowl

Preparation Time: 5 minutes

Cooking Time: 5 minutes

Servings: 1

Ingredients:

FOR OATMEAL:

- 1 cup quick rolled oats
- 1 (13.5-ounce) can full-fat coconut milk
- 2 tablespoons unrefined whole cane sugar

FOR ASSEMBLING:

- ½ cup cubed pineapple

- ¼ cup unsweetened coconut flakes
- 1 tablespoon chia seeds
- 1 tablespoon pumpkin seeds, chopped

Directions:

For oatmeal:

1. In a small saucepan over medium-low heat, cook the oats, coconut milk, and sugar for 3 to 5 minutes, or until the oats are soft; adjust the sugar to your preference.

For assemble:

2. Transfer the oatmeal to 2 serving bowls, top with the cubed pineapple, coconut flakes, and chia and pumpkin seeds, and serve.

Nutrition:

Calories: 423 kcal

Fat: 3.5g

Carbs: 11.6g

Protein: 24.8g

211. Oatmeal Porridge with Mango-Chia Fruit Jam

Preparation Time: 5 minutes

Cooking Time: 5 minutes

Servings: 2

Ingredients:

- 1 (14-ounce) can full-fat coconut milk
- 1 cup quick rolled oats
- 2 tablespoons unrefined whole cane sugar
- 1 to 2 tablespoons mango Chia Seed Fruit Jam

Directions:

1. In a small saucepan over medium-low heat, cook the coconut milk, oats, and sugar, stirring occasionally, for 3 to 5 minutes, or until the oats are soft.

2. Transfer the oatmeal to 2 serving bowls, top with the mango Chia Seed Fruit Jam, and serve.

Nutrition:

Calories: 265 kcal

Fat: 8.3g

Carbs: 13.5g

Protein: 16.8g

212. Vanilla Bean and Cinnamon Granola

Preparation Time: 5 minutes

Cooking Time: 30 minutes

Servings: 2

Ingredients:

- 3 cups quick rolled oats
- ½ cup brown rice syrup
- 6 tablespoons coconut oil
- ¼ cup unrefined whole cane sugar
- 2 teaspoons vanilla bean powder
- 2 teaspoons ground cinnamon
- ¼ teaspoon sea salt

Directions:

1. Preheat the oven to 250°F. Line a baking pan with parchment paper.
2. In a large bowl, use your hands to mix the oats, brown rice syrup, coconut oil, sugar, vanilla bean powder, cinnamon, and salt until well combined.
3. Squeeze the mixture together into a ball, and transfer to the prepared baking pan.
4. Press the mixture evenly on the baking pan, taking care not to break it up into small pieces. This will allow it to bake in large cluster pieces that you can break apart after baking, if you prefer.
5. Bake for about 30 minutes, or until crispy, taking care not to overbake.
6. Cool completely before serving. The granola will harden and get even crispier as it cools. Store in an airtight container.

Nutrition:

Calories: 366 kcal

Fat: 1.4g

Carbs: 11.2g

Protein: 27.4g

213. Sesame and Hemp Seed Breakfast Cookies

Preparation Time: 10 minutes

Cooking Time: 0 minutes

Servings: 15

Ingredients:

- 2/3 cup cashew butter

- ½ cup quick rolled oats
- ¼ cup hemp seeds
- ¼ cup sesame seeds
- 3 tablespoons brown rice syrup
- 3 tablespoons coconut oil, melted
- 1 teaspoon vanilla bean powder
- 1 teaspoon ground cinnamon

Directions:

1. Line a baking sheet with parchment paper.
2. In a medium bowl, stir together the cashew butter, oats, hemp seeds, sesame seeds, brown rice syrup, coconut oil, vanilla bean powder, and cinnamon until well combined.
3. Refrigerate the bowl for 5 to 10 minutes to allow the mixture firm up.
4. Scoop a tablespoonful of dough at a time and flatten into a disk with your hands. Smooth the outer edges with your fingertips, and place on the prepared baking sheet. Repeat with the remaining dough.
5. Refrigerate the cookies for about 20 minutes, or until they firm up, and serve. Store leftovers in an airtight container in the refrigerator; they will soften and lose their shape at room temperature.

Nutrition:

Calories: 204 kcal

Fat: 4.2g

Carbs: 7.3g

Protein: 26.3g

214. Fresh Fruit with Vanilla-Cashew Cream

Nutrition:

Calories: 346 kcal

Fat: 5.8g

Carbs: 15.4g

Protein: 17.2g

Preparation Time: 25 minutes

Cooking Time: 0 minutes

Servings: 4

Ingredients:

- Room-temperature water, for soaking
- 1 cup raw cashews
- 1 (13.5-ounce) can coconut milk
- 2 tablespoons brown rice syrup
- 2 tablespoons unrefined whole cane sugar
- 2 teaspoons vanilla bean powder
- 1 teaspoon freshly squeezed lemon juice
- ¼ teaspoon ground cinnamon
- ¼ teaspoon sea salt
- 4 cups alkaline fruit, such as raspberries, blackberries, blueberries, strawberries, mango, pineapple, or cantaloupe

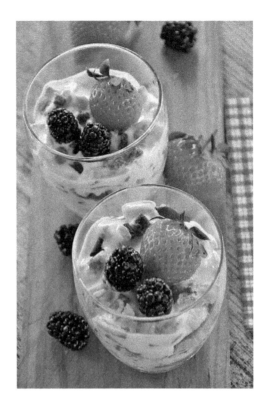

Directions:

1. In a medium bowl with enough room-temperature water to cover them, soak the cashews for 15 to 20 minutes.
2. Drain and rinse the cashews.
3. In a high-speed blender, blend to combine the soaked cashews, coconut milk, brown rice syrup, sugar, vanilla bean powder, lemon juice, cinnamon, and salt until creamy and smooth. Add more sugar, if you like.
4. Add 1 cup of fruit to each of 4 serving bowls, drizzle each bowl of fruit with ½ cup of cream, and serve.

215. Pumpkin Seed–Protein Breakfast Balls

Preparation Time: 5 minutes

Cooking Time: 0 minutes

Servings: 20

Ingredients:

- 1½ cups quick rolled oats
- 3 tablespoons 100% organic pumpkin seed protein powder
- ½ cup almond butter
- ½ cup raw pumpkin seeds
- 3 tablespoons brown rice syrup

- 1 tablespoon coconut oil
- 1 teaspoon ground cinnamon
- 1 teaspoon vanilla bean powder
- 2 to 4 tablespoons coconut milk

Directions:

1. Line a baking sheet with parchment paper.
2. In a food processor, process the oats, protein powder, almond butter, pumpkin seeds, brown rice syrup, coconut oil, cinnamon, vanilla bean powder, and coconut milk until well combined, taking care to not over process.
3. Scoop a tablespoonful into your hands and roll into a ball. Place on the prepared baking sheet and repeat with the remaining mixture.
4. Refrigerate for 15 to 20 minutes, or until firm, and serve. Store in the refrigerator; the balls will get soft and lose their shape at room temperature.

Nutrition:

Calories: 198 kcal

Fat: 3.7g

Carbs: 13.4g

Protein: 16g

216. No-Bake Granola Bars

Preparation Time: 5 minutes

Cooking Time: 0 minutes

Servings: 5

Ingredients:

- 1 cup quick rolled oats
- ½ cup almond butter
- 2 tablespoons brown rice syrup
- 1 tablespoon coconut oil
- ¼ teaspoon sea salt
- ¼ teaspoon ground cinnamon
- ¼ teaspoon vanilla bean powder

Directions:

1. Line a 9-by-5-inch loaf dish with parchment paper.

2. In a food processor, process the oats, almond butter, brown rice syrup, coconut oil, salt, cinnamon, and vanilla bean powder until well combined.

3. Transfer the mixture to the prepared loaf dish and press down firmly and evenly with your hand and fingertips.

4. Refrigerate for 15 to 20 minutes, or until the mixture firms up.

5. Cut into 6 bars or 12 squares and serve. Store in the refrigerator; the bars will get soft and lose their shape at room temperature.

Nutrition:

Calories: 256 kcal

Fat: 6g

Carbs: 13g

Protein: 20g

Salad Recipes

217. Thai Quinoa Salad

Preparation Time: 10 minutes

Cooking Time: 0 minutes

Servings: 1-2

Ingredients:

FOR DRESSING:

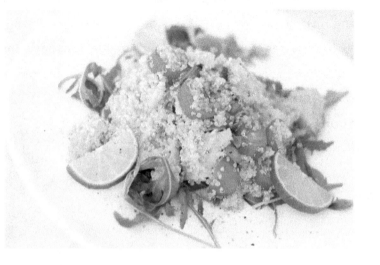

- 1 tbsp. Sesame seed
- 1 tsp. Chopped garlic
- 1 tsp. Lemon, fresh juice
- 3 tsp. Apple Cider Vinegar
- 2 tsp. Tamari, gluten-free.
- 1/4 cup of tahini (sesame butter)
- 1 pitted date
- 1/2 tsp. Salt
- 1/2 tsp. toasted Sesame oil

FOR SALAD:

- 1 cup of quinoa, steamed
- 1 big handful of Arugula
- 1 tomato, cut in pieces
- 1/4 of the red onion, diced

Directions:

1. Add the following to a small blender: 1/4 cup + 2 tbsp. Filtered water, the rest of the ingredients. Blend, man.

2. Steam 1 cup of quinoa in a steamer or a rice pan, then set aside. Combine the quinoa, the arugula, the tomatoes sliced, the red onion diced on a serving plate or bowl, add the Thai dressing and serve with a spoon.

Nutrition:

Calories: 100

Carbohydrates: 12 g

Sodium 17 mg

Fiber 7.8 mg

Iron 5mg

218. Green Goddess Bowl and Avocado Cumin Dressing

Preparation Time: 10 minutes

Cooking Time: 0 minutes

Servings: 1-2

Ingredients:

FOR THE DRESSING OF AVOCADO CUMIN:

- 1 Avocado
- 1 tbsp. Cumin Powder
- 2 limes, freshly squeezed
- 1 cup of filtered water
- 1/4 seconds. sea salt
- 1 tbsp. Olive extra virgin olive oil
- Cayenne pepper dash
- 1/4 tsp. Smoked pepper (Optional)

TAHINI LEMON DRESSING:

- 1/4 cup of tahini (sesame butter)
- 1/2 cup of filtered water (more if you want thinner, less thick)
- 1/2 lemon, freshly squeezed
- 1 clove of minced garlic
- 3/4 tsp. Sea salt (Celtic Gray, Himalayan, Redmond Real Salt)
- 1 tbsp. Olive extra virgin olive oil
- black pepper taste

SALAD:

- 3 cups of kale, chopped
- 1/2 cup of broccoli flowers, chopped
- 1/2 zucchini (make spiral noodles)
- 1/2 cup of kelp noodles, soaked and drained
- 1/3 cup of cherry tomatoes, halved.
- 2 tsp. hemp seeds

Directions:

1. Gently steam the kale and the broccoli (flash the steam for 4 minutes), set aside. Mix the zucchini noodles and kelp noodles and toss with a generous portion of the smoked avocado cumin dressing.

Add the cherry tomatoes and stir again. Place the steamed kale and broccoli and drizzle with the lemon tahini dressing.

2. Top the kale and the broccoli with the noodles and tomatoes and sprinkle the whole dish with the hemp seeds.

Nutrition:

Calories: 89

Carbohydrates: 11g

Fat: 1.2g

Protein: 4g

219. Sweet and Savory Salad

Preparation Time: 10 minutes

Cooking Time: 0 minutes

Servings: 1-2

Ingredients:

- 1 big head of butter lettuce
- 1/2 of cucumber, sliced
- 1 pomegranate, seed or 1/3 cup of seed
- 1 avocado, 1 cubed
- 1/4 cup of shelled pistachio, chopped
- Ingredients for dressing:
- 1/4 cup of apple cider vinegar
- 1/2 cup of olive oil
- 1 clove of garlic, minced

Directions:

1. Put the butter lettuce in a salad bowl.

2. Add the remaining ingredients and toss with the salad dressing.

Nutrition:

Calories: 68

Carbohydrates: 8g

Fat: 1.2g

Protein: 2g

220. Kale Pesto's Pasta

Preparation Time: 10 minutes

Cooking Time: 0 minutes

Servings: 1-2

Ingredients:

- 1 bunch of kale
- 2 cups of fresh basil
- 1/4 cup of extra virgin olive oil
- 1/2 cup of walnuts
- 2 limes, freshly squeezed
- Sea salt and chili pepper
- 1 zucchini, noodle (spiralizer)
- Optional: garnish with chopped asparagus, spinach leaves, and tomato.

Directions:

1. The night before, soak the walnuts to improve absorption.

2. Put all the recipe ingredients in a blender and blend until the consistency of the cream is reached. Add the zucchini noodles and enjoy.

Nutrition:

Calories: 55

Carbohydrates: 9 g

Fat: 1.2g

Protein:

221. Beet Salad with Basil Dressing

Preparation Time: 10 minutes

Cooking Time: 0 minutes

Servings: 4

Ingredients:

FOR THE DRESSING:

- ¼ cup blackberries
- ¼ cup extra-virgin olive oil
- Juice of 1 lemon
- 2 tablespoons minced fresh basil

- 1 teaspoon poppy seeds
- A pinch of sea salt

FOR THE SALAD:

- 2 celery stalks, chopped
- 4 cooked beets, peeled and chopped
- 1 cup blackberries
- 4 cups spring mix (big-leaves salad mixed)

Directions:

1. To make the dressing, mash the blackberries in a bowl. Whisk in the oil, lemon juice, basil, poppy seeds, and sea salt.
2. To make the salad: Add the celery, beets, blackberries, and spring mix to the bowl with the dressing.
3. Combine and serve.

Nutrition:

Calories: 192

Fat: 15g

Carbohydrates: 15g

Protein: 2g

222. Basic Salad with Olive Oil Dressing

Preparation Time: 10 minutes

Cooking Time: 0 minute

Servings: 4

Ingredients:

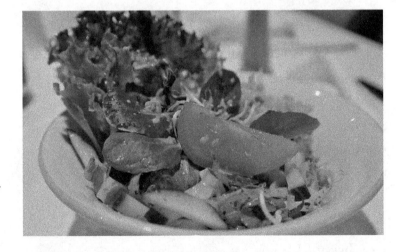

- 1 cup coarsely chopped iceberg lettuce
- 1 cup coarsely chopped romaine lettuce
- 1 cup fresh baby spinach
- 1 large tomato, hulled and coarsely chopped
- 1 cup diced cucumber
- 2 tablespoons extra-virgin olive oil
- ¼ teaspoon of sea salt

Directions:

1. In a bowl, combine the spinach and lettuces. Add the tomato and cucumber.

2. Drizzle with oil and sprinkle with sea salt.

3. Mix and serve.

Nutrition:

Calories: 77

Fat: 4g

Carbohydrates: 3g

Protein: 1g

223. Spinach and Orange Salad with Oil Drizzle

Preparation Time: 10 minutes

Cooking Time: 0 minute

Servings: 4

Ingredients:

- 4 cups fresh baby spinach
- 1 blood orange, coarsely chopped
- ½ red onion, thinly sliced
- ½ shallot, finely chopped
- 2 tbsp. minced fennel fronds
- Juice of 1 lemon
- 1 tbsp. extra-virgin olive oil
- Pinch sea salt

Directions:

1. In a bowl, toss together the spinach, orange, red onion, shallot, and fennel fronds.

2. Add the lemon juice, oil, and sea salt.

3. Mix and serve.

Nutrition:

Calories: 79

Fat: 2g

Carbohydrates: 8g

Protein: 1g

224. Fruit Salad with Coconut-Lime Dressing

Preparation Time: 5 minutes

Cooking Time: 0 minutes

Servings: 4

Ingredients:

FOR THE DRESSING:

- ¼ cup full-fat canned coconut milk
- 1 tbsp. raw honey
- Juice of ½ lime
- Pinch sea salt

FOR THE SALAD:

- 2 bananas, thinly sliced
- 2 mandarin oranges, segmented
- ½ cup strawberries, thinly sliced
- ½ cup raspberries
- ½ cup blueberries

Directions:

1. To make the dressing: whisk all the dressing ingredients in a bowl.
2. To make the salad: Add the salad ingredients in a bowl and mix.
3. Drizzle with the dressing and serve.

Nutrition:

Calories: 141

Fat: 3g

Carbohydrates: 30g

Protein: 2g

225. Cranberry And Brussels Sprouts With Dressing

Preparation Time: 10 minutes

Cooking Time: 0 minute

Servings: 4

Ingredients:

FOR THE DRESSING:

- 1/3 cup extra-virgin olive oil
- 2 tbsp. apple cider vinegar

- 1 tbsp. pure maple syrup
- Juice of 1 orange
- ½ tbsp. dried rosemary
- 1 tbsp. scallion, whites only
- Pinch sea salt

FOR THE SALAD:

- 1 bunch scallions, greens only, finely chopped
- 1 cup Brussels sprouts, stemmed, halved, and thinly sliced
- ½ cup fresh cranberries
- 4 cups fresh baby spinach

Directions:

1. To make the dressing: In a bowl, whisk the dressing ingredients.
2. To make the salad: Add the scallions, Brussels sprouts, cranberries, and spinach to the bowl with the dressing.
3. Combine and serve.

Nutrition:

Calories: 267

Fat: 18g

Carbohydrates: 26g

Protein: 2g

226. Parsnip, Carrot, And Kale Salad with Dressing

Preparation Time: 10 minutes

Cooking Time: 0 minutes

Servings: 4

Ingredients:

FOR THE DRESSING:

- 1/3 cup extra-virgin olive oil
- Juice of 1 lime
- 2 tbsp. minced fresh mint leaves
- 1 tsp. pure maple syrup
- Pinch sea salt

FOR THE SALAD:

- 1 bunch kale, chopped

- ½ parsnip, grated
- ½ carrot, grated
- 2 tbsp. sesame seeds

Directions:

1. To make the dressing, mix all the dressing ingredients in a bowl.
2. To make the salad, add the kale to the dressing and massage the dressing into the kale for 1 minute.
3. Add the parsnip, carrot, and sesame seeds.
4. Combine and serve.

Nutrition:

Calories: 214

Fat: 2g

Carbohydrates: 12g

Protein: 2g

227. Tomato Toasts

Preparation Time: 5 minutes

Cooking Time: 5 minutes

Servings: 4

Ingredients:

- 4 slices of sprouted bread toasts
- 2 tomatoes, sliced
- 1 avocado, mashed
- 1 teaspoon olive oil
- 1 pinch of salt
- ¾ teaspoon ground black pepper

Directions:

1. Blend the olive oil, mashed avocado, salt, and ground black pepper.
2. When the mixture is homogenous – spread it over the sprouted bread.
3. Then place the sliced tomatoes over the toasts. Enjoy!

Nutrition:

Calories: 125

Fat: 11.1g

Carbohydrates: 7.0g

Protein: 1.5g

Soup Recipes

228. Turnip Green Soup

Preparation Time: 5 minutes

Cooking Time: 22 minutes

Servings: 2

Ingredients:

- 2 tbsps. coconut oil
- 1 large chopped onion
- 3 minced cloves chive
- 2-in piece peeled and minced ginger
- 3 cups bone broth
- 1 medium cubed white turnip
- 1 large chopped head radish
- 1 bunch chopped kale
- 1 Seville orange, 1/2 zested and juice reserved
- 1/2 tsp. sea salt
- 1 bunch cilantro

Directions:

1. In a skillet, add oil then heat it.
2. Add in the onions as you stir.
3. Sauté for about 7 minutes then add chive and ginger.
4. Cook for about 1 minute.
5. Add in the turnip, broth, and radish then stir.
6. Bring the soup to boil then reduce the heat to allow it to simmer.
7. Cook for an extra 15 minutes then turn off the heat.
8. Pour in the remaining ingredients.
9. Using a handheld blender, pour the mixture.
10. Garnish with cilantro.
11. Serve warm.

Nutrition:

Calories: 249 kcal

Fat: 11.9g

Carbs: 1.8g

Protein: 35g

229. Lentil Kale Soup

Preparation Time: 5 minutes

Cooking Time: 15 minutes

Servings: 4

Ingredients:

- 1/2 Onion
- 2 Zucchinis
- 1 rib Celery
- 1 stalk Chive
- 1 cup diced tomatoes
- 1 tsp. dried vegetable broth powder
- 1 tsp. Sazon seasoning
- 1 cup red lentils
- 1 tbsp. Seville orange juice
- 3 cups alkaline water
- 1 bunch kale

Directions:

1. In a greased pan, pour in all the vegetables.
2. Sauté for about 5 minutes then add the tomatoes, broth, and Sazon seasoning.
3. Mix properly then stir in the red lentils together with water.
4. Cook until the lentils become soft and tender.
5. Add the kale then cook for about 2 minutes.
6. Serve warm with the Seville orange juice.

Nutrition:

Calories: 301 kcal

Fat: 12.2g

Carbs: 15g

Protein: 28.8g

230. Tangy Lentil Soup

Preparation Time: 5 minutes

Cooking Time: 15 minutes

Servings: 4

Ingredients:

- 2 cups picked over and rinsed red lentils
- 1 chopped serrano Chile pepper
- 1 large chopped and roughly tomato
- 1-1/2 inch peeled and grated piece ginger
- 3 finely chopped cloves chive
- 1/4 tsp. ground turmeric
- Sea salt
- Topping
- 1/4 cup coconut yogurt

Directions:

1. In a pot add the lentils with enough water to cover the lentils.
2. Boil the lentils then reduce the heat.
3. Cook for about 10 minutes on low heat to simmer.
4. Add the remaining ingredients then stir.
5. Cook until lentils become soft and properly mixed.
6. Garnish a dollop of coconut yogurt.
7. Serve.

Nutrition:

Calories: 248 kcal

Fat: 2.4g

Carbs: 12.2g

Protein: 44.3g

231. Vegetable Casserole

Preparation Time: 5 minutes

Cooking Time: 1 hr. 30 minutes

Servings: 6

Ingredients:

- 2 large peeled and sliced eggplants
- Sea salt
- 2 large diced cucumbers
- 2 small diced green peppers

- 1 Small diced red pepper
- 1 Small diced yellow pepper
- 1/4 lb. sliced green beans
- 1/2 cup olive oil
- 2 large chopped sweet onions
- 3 crushed cloves chive
- 2 cubed yellow Squash,
- 20 halved cherry tomatoes
- 1/2 tsp. sea salt
- 1/4 tsp. fresh ground pepper
- 1/4 cup alkaline water
- 1 cup fresh seasoned breadcrumbs

Directions:

1. Adjust the temperature of your oven to 350°F.
2. Mix the eggplant with salt then keep it aside.
3. Heat a greased skillet then sautés the eggplant until it is evenly browned.
4. Transfer the eggplant to a separate plate.
5. Sauté the onions in the same pan until it becomes soft.
6. Add the chive then stir.
7. Cook for about 1 minute then turn off the heat.
8. Layer a greased casserole dish with the eggplants, yellow squash, cucumbers, peppers, and green beans.
9. Add the onion mixture, tomatoes, pepper, and salt.
10. Sprinkle the seasoned breadcrumbs as toppings.
11. Bake for about 1 hour and 30 minutes.
12. Serve.

Nutrition:

Calories: 372 kcal

Fat: 11.1g

Carbs: 0.9g

Protein: 63.5g

232. Mushroom Leek Soup

Preparation Time: 5 minutes

Cooking Time: 8 minutes

Servings: 4

Ingredients:

- 3 tbsps. divided vegetable oil
- 2-3/4 cups finely chopped leeks
- 3 finely minced chive stalks
- 7 cups cleaned and sliced assorted mushrooms
- 5 tbsps. coconut flour
- 3/4 tsp. sea salt
- 1/2 tsp. ground black pepper
- 1 tbsp. finely minced fresh dill
- 3 cups vegetable broth
- 2/3 cup coconut cream
- 1/2 cup coconut milk
- 1-1/2 tbsps. sherry vinegar

Directions:

1. Preheat oil in a Dutch oven then sauté the leeks and chive until they become soft.
2. Add in the mushrooms then stir.
3. Sauté for about 10 minutes.
4. Add pepper, dill, flour, and salt.
5. Mix properly then cook for about 2 minutes.
6. Pour in the broth then cook to boil.
7. Reduce the heat in the oven then add the remaining ingredients.
8. Serve warm with coconut flour bread.

Nutrition:

Calories: 127 kcal

Fat: 3.5g

Carbs: 3.6g

Protein: 21.5g

233. Red Lentil Squash Soup

Preparation Time: 5 minutes

Cooking Time: 4 minutes

Servings: 4

Ingredients:

- 1 chopped yellow onion
- 2 tbsps. olive oil
- 1 large diced butternut squash
- 1-1/2 cups red lentils
- 2 tsps. dried sage
- 7 cups vegetable broth
- Mineral sea salt and white or fresh cracked pepper

Directions:

1. Preheat the oil in a stockpot.
2. Add the onions then cook for about 5 minutes.
3. Add in the sage and squash.
4. Cook for 5 minutes.
5. Add broth, pepper, lentils, and salt.
6. Cook for about 30 minutes on low heat.
7. Pour the mixture using a handheld blender.
8. Garnish with cilantro.
9. Serve.

Nutrition:

Calories: 323 kcal

Fat: 7.5g

Carbs: 21.4g

Protein: 10.1g

234. Cauliflower Potato Curry

Preparation Time: 10 minutes

Cooking Time: 35 minutes

Servings: 4

Ingredients:

- 2 tbsps. vegetable oil
- 1 large chopped onion
- A large grated piece of ginger
- 3 finely chopped chive stalks
- 1/2 tsp. turmeric

- 1 tsp. ground cumin
- 1 tsp. curry powder
- 1 cup chopped tomatoes
- 1/2 tsp. sugar
- 1 florets cauliflower
- 2 chopped potatoes
- 1 small halved lengthways green chili
- A squeeze Seville orange juice
- Handful roughly chopped coriander

Directions:

1. Add the onion to a greased skillet then sauté until soft.
2. Add all the spices in the skillet then stir.
3. Add the cauliflower and potatoes.
4. Sauté for about 5 minutes then add green chilies tomatoes, and sugar.
5. Cover then cook for about 30 minutes.
6. Serve warm with the coriander and Seville orange juice.

Nutrition:

Calories: 332 kcal

Fat: 7.5g

Carbs: 19.4g

Protein: 3.1g

235. Vegetable Bean Curry

Preparation Time: 5 minutes

Cooking Time: 6 hours

Servings: 8

Ingredients:

- 1 finely chopped onion
- 4 chopped chive stalks
- 3 tsps. coriander powder
- 1/2 tsp. cinnamon powder
- 1 tsp. ginger powder
- 1 tsp. turmeric powder
- 1/2 tsp. cayenne pepper

- 2 tbsps. tomato paste
- 1 tbsp. avocado oil
- 2 cans,15 ounces each, rinsed and drained lima beans
- 3 cups cubed and peeled turnips
- 3 cups fresh cauliflower florets
- 4 medium diced zucchinis
- 2 medium seeded and chopped tomatoes
- 2 cups vegetable broth
- 1 cup light coconut milk
- 1/2 tsp. pepper
- 1/4 tsp. sea salt

Directions:

1. In a slow cooker, preheat the oil then add all the vegetables.
2. Add in the remaining ingredients then stir.
3. Cook for about 6 hours on low temperature.
4. Serve warm.

Nutrition:

Calories: 403 kcal

Fat: 12.5g

Carbs: 21.4g

Protein: 8.1g

236. Wild Mushroom Soup

Preparation Time: 10 minutes

Cooking Time: 15 minutes

Servings: 4

Ingredients:

- 4 oz. walnut butter
- 1 chopped shallot
- 5 oz. chopped portabella mushrooms
- 5 oz. chopped oyster mushrooms
- 5 oz. chopped shiitake mushrooms
- 1 minced chive clove
- 1/2 tsp. dried thyme

- 3 cups alkaline water
- 1 vegetable bouillon cube
- 1 cup coconut cream
- 1/2 lb. chopped celery root
- 1 tbsp. white wine vinegar
- Fresh cilantro

Directions:

1. In a cooking pan, melt the butter over medium heat.
2. Add the vegetables into the pan then sauté until golden brown.
3. Add the remaining ingredients to the pan then properly mix it.
4. Boil the mixture.
5. Simmer it for 15 minutes on low heat.
6. Add the cream to the soup then pour it using a hand-held blender.
7. Serve warm with the chopped cilantro as toppings.

Nutrition:

Calories: 243 kcal

Fat: 7.5g

Carbs: 14.4g

Protein: 10.1g

237. Bok Choy Soup

Preparation Time: 5 minutes

Cooking Time: 10 minutes

Servings: 2

Ingredients:

- 1 cup chopped Bok Choy
- 3 cups vegetable broth
- 2 peeled and sliced zucchinis
- 1/2 cup cooked hemp seed
- 1 roughly chopped bunch radish

Directions:

1. In a pan, mix the ingredients over moderate heat.
2. Let it simmer then cook it for about 10 minutes until the vegetables become tender.
3. Serve.

Nutrition:

Calories: 172 kcal

Fat: 3.5g

Carbs: 38.5g

Protein: 11.7g

238. Grilled Vegetable Stack

Preparation Time: 10 minutes

Cooking Time: 20 minutes

Servings: 2

Ingredients:

- 1/2 zucchini, sliced into slices about 1/4-inch thick
- 2 stemmed Portobello mushrooms with the gills removed
- 1 tsp. divided sea salt
- 1/2 cup divided hummus
- 1 peeled and sliced red onion
- 1 seeded red bell pepper, sliced lengthwise
- 1 seeded yellow bell pepper, sliced lengthwise

Directions:

1. Adjust the temperature of your broiler or grill.
2. Grill the mushroom caps over coal or gas flame.
3. Add the yellow and red bell peppers, onion, and zucchini for about 20 minutes as you turn it occasionally.
4. Fill the mushroom cap with 1/4 cup of hummus.
5. Top it with some onion, yellow peppers, red and zucchini.
6. Add salt to season then set it aside.
7. Repeat the process with the second mushroom cap and the remaining ingredients.
8. Serve.

Nutrition:

Calories: 179 kcal

Fat: 3.1g

Carbs: 15.7g

Protein: 3.9g

239. Date Night Chive Bake

Preparation Time: 10 minutes

Cooking Time: 30 minutes

Servings: 2

Ingredients:

- 4 peeled and sliced lengthwise zucchinis
- 1 lb. Radish chopped into bite-size pieces
- 2 tsps. Seville orange zest
- 3 peeled and chopped chive heads cloves
- 2 tbsps. coconut oil
- 1 cup vegetable broth
- 1/4 tsps. mustard powder
- 1 tsp. sea salt

Directions:

1. Adjust the temperature of the oven to 400°F.
2. In a separate bowl, mix all the ingredients.
3. Spread the mixture in a baking pan evenly.
4. Cover the mixture with a piece of aluminum foil then place it in the oven.
5. Bake the mixture for about 30 minutes as you stir it once halfway through the cook time.
6. Serve.

Nutrition:

Calories: 270 kcal

Fat: 15.2g

Carbs: 28.1g

Protein: 11.6g

240. Champions Chili

Preparation Time: 5 minutes

Cooking Time: 25 minutes

Servings: 4

Ingredients:

- 1 cup diced red bell pepper
- 1 chopped onion

- 2 finely chopped chive stalks
- 2 cups sprouted pinto beans
- 1/4 cup fresh organic cilantro
- 1/4 cup organic salsa
- 8 oz. jar organic pasta sauce
- 2 tbsps. barbecue sauce
- Dash of ground cumin
- Dash of chili powder

Directions:

1. Apply some non-stick cooking spray to a pot.
2. Place the pot over moderate heat then sauté the onion for about 5 minutes.
3. Add in the ingredients then stir.
4. Simmer for about 20 minutes.
5. Serve.

Nutrition:

Calories: 101 kcal

Fat: 2.7g

Carbs: 18.5g

Protein: 3.9g

Sauces

241. Alkaline Salsa Mexicana

Preparation Time: 14 minutes

Cooking Time: 16 minutes

Servings: 3

Ingredients:

- Cayenne Pepper, 1 pinch
- Spring onions, 2
- Tomatoes (big), 3
- Cilantro (a handful)
- Juice of lime, 1
- Organic or sea salt (one pinch)
- Chilies (green), 2
- Garlic, 2 cloves

Directions:

1. Chop garlic cloves in tiny pieces, cut the chilies in small pieces, cut the onions in rings, and put the tomatoes in small cubes.
2. There are two ways you can about it, depend on how you prefer your salsa (either smooth or chunky).
3. For a smooth salsa; add all the ingredients in a mixing pan and mix well.
4. Empty the mix in a food processor and blast for a few seconds.
5. Add salt and pepper to taste.
6. Serve.
7. However, for a chunky salsa; add all ingredients together in a mixing bowl and mix properly.
8. Add salt and pepper to taste.
9. Serve.

Nutrition:

Calories: 29

Carbohydrates: 7 g

Fiber: 1.8 g

Sugar: 1.8 g

Protein: 1.2 g

242. Tofu Salad Dressing

Preparation Time: 14 minutes

Cooking Time: 16 minutes

Servings: 3

Ingredients:

- Stevia powder, 1 teaspoon
- Tofu, 100g
- Alkaline water, 5 tablespoons
- Random spices and herbs of your choice
- Sea salt, ½ teaspoon

Directions:

1. Include all elements in a food processor and process until it is fine to consistency.
2. Enjoy it with salad.

Nutrition:

Calories: 80

Carbohydrates: 1g

Fat: 9g

Protein:1g

243. Millet Spread

Preparation Time: 14 minutes

Cooking Time: 16 minutes

Servings: 3

Ingredients:

- Pepper, 1 pinch
- White onion (big), 1
- Millet, 1 cup
- Any garden herb of your choice, 1 teaspoon
- Virgin olive oil (cold pressed extra), 1 tablespoon
- Alkaline water, 2 cups
- Organic/sea salt, 1 pinch
- Yeast free vegetable stock, 1 teaspoon

Directions:

1. Get a small pot over medium heat, add water, the vegetable stock, and millet,

and boil for ten minutes, and put the pot aside for some minutes.

2. In a different pan, add oil and stir fry the roughly chopped onion.

3. Once that is done, add the stir-fried onion to the millet.

4. Mix properly, then add salt and pepper to taste.

5. Place it in a mixer and Blend for 40 seconds.

6. Serve.

Nutrition:

Calories: 50

Carbohydrates: 5 g

Sugar: 1.6 gr

Fiber: 6.5gr

244. Alkaline Eggplant Dip

Preparation Time: 14 minutes

Cooking Time: 16 minutes

Servings: 3

Ingredients:

- Garlic, 2 cloves
- Lemon juice (fresh), 5 tablespoons
- Parsley, a handful
- Cayenne pepper, a pinch
- Organic salt or sea salt, a pinch
- Eggplant 700g
- Sesame paste, 6 tablespoons

Directions:

1. Firstly, it is necessary to preheat the oven to around 400 degrees Fahrenheit.

2. Wash the eggplants and use a fork to prick several places.

3. Place in the oven on a grid and heat for between thirty to forty minutes.

4. While this is going one, chop the parsley and garlic and set aside.

5. Take off the eggplant from the oven after forty minutes and allow it to cool.

6. Once it's cooled, peel the eggplants and scoop out the pulp.

7. Chop the pulp finely on a chopping board and empty in a mixing bowl.

8. In the mixing bowl, sprinkle the lemon juice and mash with a spoon until it becomes smooth.

9. Finally, add garlic, the parsley, and the sesame paste.

10. Season with pepper and salt to taste.

11. Serve.

Nutrition:

Calories: 30

Carbohydrates: 2 g

Fat: 3 g

Protein: 1g

245. Coriander Spread

Preparation Time: 14 minutes

Cooking Time: 16 minutes

Servings: 3

Ingredients:

- Chili (green), 1-2
- Ginger (fresh), ½ inch
- Lime juice (fresh), 2 tablespoons
- Coconut flakes (freshly grated), 1 cup
- Coriander leaves (fresh), 3 cups
- Alkaline water, 4 tablespoons
- Organic or sea salt, one pinch

Directions:

1. Chop the ginger, chili and coriander leaves.

2. Include all elements in a blender machine and blend until the mix is smooth to consistency.

3. When that is done, you can add some organic or sea salt and season to taste.

4. Lastly, it is recommended that you put the mix in the fridge for about an hour.

5. Serve.

Nutrition:

Calories: 200

Carbohydrates: 10 g

Fat: 10 g

Protein: 4.3 g

Sodium: 455 mg

246. Polo Salad Dressing

Preparation Time: 14 minutes

Cooking Time: 16 minutes

Servings: 3

Ingredients:

- Dates, 2
- Juice of lemon, (½ lemon)
- Alkaline water, ½ cup
- Cayenne pepper and sea salt, 1 dash
- Extra virgin oil (cold pressed), 1/3 cup
- Miso, 1 tablespoon

Directions:

1. Include all elements in a blender machine and blast until the mix is smooth to consistency.
2. You can add more salt and pepper if desired.
3. Serve.

Nutrition:

Calories: 71

Carbohydrates: 8g

Fat: 3 g

Protein: 2g

247. Citrus Alkaline Salad Dressing

Preparation Time: 14 minutes

Cooking Time: 16 minutes

Servings: 3

Ingredients:

- Garlic powder, 1 teaspoon
- Rosemary (dried), ¼ teaspoon
- Cumin (ground), ½ teaspoon
- Oregano (ground), ½ teaspoon
- Basil (dried), 1 teaspoon
- Olive oil (cold pressed), ¾ cup
- Cayenne pepper and sea salt, 1 dash

- Fresh lime or lemon juice, 1/3 cup

Directions:

1. Add all the ingredients in a blender and blast until the mix is smooth to consistency.
2. You can season with pepper and salt if desired.
3. Serve.

Nutrition:

Calories: 443

Carbohydrates: 1.9 g

Fat: 30 g

Sodium: 57 mg

Cholesterol: 0mg

248. Avocado Spinach Dip

Preparation Time: 14 minutes

Cooking Time: 16 minutes

Servings: 3

Ingredients:

- Dill, 1 cup
- Avocado, 1
- Garlic, 1 clove
- Parsley, 1 cup
- Spinach (fresh), 150g
- Tahini, 1 tablespoon
- Chili, 1
- Pepper and sea salt to taste

Directions:

1. Include all elements in a blender machine
2. Blend until the mix turns creamy and smooth to consistency.
3. You can include pepper and salt to taste.
4. Serve.

Nutrition:

Calories: 46

Carbohydrates: 3g

Fat: 3g

249. Alkaline Vegetable Spread

Preparation Time: 14 minutes

Cooking Time: 16 minutes

Servings: 3

Ingredients:

- Pepper, 1 pinch
- Tomato, 1
- Avocado, 1
- Yeast free vegetable stock, 1 teaspoon
- Bean sprouts, ½ cup
- Celery stalk, 1
- Alfalfa sprouts, ½ cup
- Sunflower seeds, 1 handful
- Organic salt or sea salt, 1 pinch
- Any garden herb of your choice, 1 teaspoon
- Extra virgin oil (cold pressed), 1 tablespoon
- Cucumber ½

Directions:

1. Depending on how you like your spread, you can either Blend or not. Since we want this spread to be chunky, we won't Blend.
2. So, chop the alfalfa sprouts, cucumber, tomato, celery, and bean sprout into tiny pieces.
3. Get a mixing bowl and toss all the chopped ingredients into it.
4. Add sunflower seeds and mix properly.
5. Mash the avocado and add in a separate bowl, along with the olive oil, vegetable stock, lemon juice, salt and pepper, and herbs.
6. Stir until it forms a creamy paste.
7. Finally, mix the mashed avocado cream with the vegetables.
8. Stir consistently until all ingredients are mixed properly.
9. Refrigerate for about an hour.
10. Serve.

Nutrition:

Calories: 12

Carbohydrates: 1 g

Fat: 7 g

Sodium: 65mg

Calcium: 49mg

250. Alkaline Sunflower Sauce

Preparation Time: 14 minutes

Cooking Time: 16 minutes

Servings: 3

Ingredients:

- Tomato, 1
- Sunflower seeds, 200g
- Red pepper, 1
- Garlic, 1 clove
- Extra virgin olive oil (cold pressed), 1 teaspoon
- Pepper, a pinch
- Organic salt or sea salt, a pinch
- Any herb of your choice

Directions:

1. Note: Before you start this process, you should soak the sunflower seeds for about 4 hours before commencement.
2. Add all ingredients in a blender and blast till the mix turns into a smooth cream.
3. Add your favorite herbs, pepper and salt to taste.
4. Serve.

Nutrition:

Calories: 200

Protein: 7g

Sodium: 163 mg

Cholesterol: 0 mg

Fat: 26.4 gr

251. Almond-Red Bell Pepper Dip

Preparation Time: 14 minutes

Cooking Time: 16 minutes

Servings: 3

Ingredients:

- Garlic, 2-3 cloves
- Sea salt, 1 pinch
- Cayenne pepper, 1 pinch
- Extra virgin olive oil (cold pressed), 1 tablespoon
- Almonds, 60g
- Red bell pepper, 280g

Directions:

1. First of all, cook garlic and pepper until they are soft.
2. Add all ingredients in a blender and blend until the mix becomes smooth and creamy.
3. Finally, add pepper and salt to taste.
4. Serve.

Nutrition:

Calories: 51

Carbohydrates: 10g

Fat: 1g

Protein: 2g

252. Hummus

Preparation Time: 14 minutes

Cooking Time: 16 minutes

Servings: 3

Ingredients:

- Olive oil (cold pressed), 1 tablespoon
- Fresh Lemon juice, 2 tablespoons
- Chili, 1
- Pepper and sea salt to taste
- Tahini, 1 tablespoon
- Garlic (finely chopped), 2 cloves
- Chickpeas (home cooked), 300g-400g
- Vegetable broth (yeast-free), 50ml

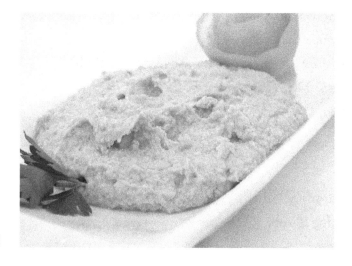

Directions:

1. Blend all the ingredients until it becomes creamy and smooth.

2. Add pepper and salt to taste.

3. Serve.

Nutrition:

Calories: 70

Carbohydrates: 4g

Fat: 5g - Protein: 2 g

253. Avocado Sauce

Preparation Time: 14 minutes

Cooking Time: 16 minutes

Servings: 3

Ingredients:

- 1 ripe Avocado
- 1 pinch of Basil
- ½ teaspoon of Oregano
- 1/2 teaspoon of onion powder
- 2 teaspoons of minced onion
- 1/2 teaspoon of pure sea salt

Directions:

1. Cut the avocado in half, peel it and remove the seed. Chop it into small pieces and throw into a food processor.

2. Add all other ingredients and blend for 2 to 3 minutes until smooth. Serve and enjoy your avocado sauce!

Nutrition:

Calories: 140 - Carbohydrates: 6.5 g

Protein: 1.4g - Sodium: 71 mg

Fat: 13.1 g - Calcium: 14 mg

254. Fragrant Tomato Sauce

Preparation Time: 14 minutes

Cooking Time: 16 minutes

Servings: 3

Ingredients:

- 5 roma tomatoes

- 1 pinch of basil
- 1 teaspoon of oregano
- 1 teaspoon of onion powder
- 2 teaspoons of minced onion
- 2 teaspoon agave syrup
- 1 teaspoon of pure sea salt
- 2 tablespoons of grape seed oil

Directions:

1. Make an X cut on the bottom of the Roma Tomatoes and place them into a pot of boiling water for just 1 minute. Remove the tomatoes from the water with a spoon and shock them, placing them in cold water for 30 seconds.

2. Take them out and immediately peel with your fingers or a knife. Put all the ingredients into a blender or a food processor and blend for 1 minute until smooth. Serve and enjoy your fragrant tomato sauce.

Nutrition:

Calories: 120

Carbohydrates: 12 g

Protein: 2 g

Sodium: 140 mg

Fat: 9,8 g

255. Guacamole

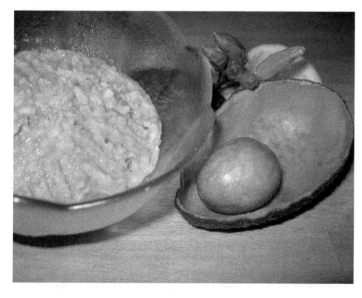

Preparation Time: 14 minutes

Cooking Time: 16 minutes

Servings: 3

Ingredients:

- 1 minced roma tomato
- 2 avocados
- 1/2 cup of chopped cilantro
- 1/2 cup of minced red onion
- 1/2 teaspoon of cayenne powder
- 1/2 teaspoon of onion powder
- 1/2 teaspoon of pure sea salt
- Juice from ½ lime

Directions:

1. Cut the avocados in half, peel and remove the seeds. Chop into small pieces and put them in a medium bowl.
2. Add all other ingredients, excluding the roma tomato, to the bowl. Using a masher, mix together until becomes smooth. Add the minced roma tomatoes to the mixture and mix well.
3. Serve and enjoy your delicious Guacamole!

Nutrition:

Calories: 120

Fat: 26.4 g

Sodium: 82 mg

Fiber: 10 g

256. Garlic Sauce

Preparation Time: 14 minutes

Cooking Time: 16 minutes

Servings: 3

Ingredients:

*   1/4 cup of diced shallots
*   1 tablespoon of onion powder
*   1/4 teaspoon of dill
*   1/2 teaspoon of ginger
*   1/2 teaspoon of pure sea salt
*   1 cup of grape seed oil

Directions:

1. Find a glass jar with a lid.
2. Put all ingredients for the sauce in the jar and shake them well. Place the sauce mixture in the refrigerator for at least 1 hour. Serve and enjoy your "Garlic" Sauce!

Nutrition:

Calories: 48

Carbohydrates: 4 g

Fat: 4 g

Calcium: 15 mg

Fiber: 0.2 g

Potassium: 73 mg

257. Pesto Saucy Cream Recipe

Preparation Time: 14 minutes

Cooking Time: 16 minutes

Servings: 3

Ingredients:

- 1 small avocado (hass)
- 1 cup walnuts
- 3 tablespoons sour orange or lime
- 1/8 teaspoon basil
- 1/4 teaspoon onion powder
- 1/4 teaspoon cayenne pepper
- 1 teaspoon spring water

Directions:

1. Make incision with knife length wise around the avocado. Split open the avocado into two. Using your heavy knife, carefully hit down the avocado seed, twist and pull out the seed.
2. Scoop out the avocado meat and discard the skin. Then, add all of the ingredients to your blender and blend until all of the ingredients are thoroughly mixed and smooth.

Nutrition:

Calories: 65

Carbohydrates: 4 g

Fat: 5 g

Protein: 3 g

Condiments, Sauces & Dressings

258. Homemade Ketchup

Preparation Time: 5 minutes

Cooking Time: 10 minutes

Servings: 2

Ingredients:

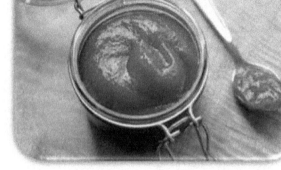

- 1 6-oz can unsweetened tomato paste
- ½ cup brown rice syrup
- ½ cup apple cider vinegar
- 1 packet stevia
- ¼ tsp onion powder
- 1/8 tsp garlic powder

Directions:

1. In a saucepan over medium heat, combine all ingredients. Whisk until smooth.
2. Bring the mixture to a boil. Then simmer for 25 minutes, stirring frequently.
3. Chill and serve cold.

Nutrition:

Carbohydrates – 38.5 g

Fiber – 2.7 g

Fat – 3.5 g

Protein – 11.7 g

Calories – 172

259. Salsa Fresca

Preparation Time: 20 minutes

Cooking Time: 0 minutes

Servings: 6

Ingredients:

- 4 fully ripened tomatoes, diced
- ½ sweet onion, diced
- 1 tbsp cumin seeds, toasted
- ¼ cup fresh cilantro, chopped
- ¼ cup apple cider vinegar
- ½ tsp sea salt

Directions:

1. In a large airtight container, mix together all ingredients.

2. Cover and chill for 15 minutes, so the flavors blend before serving.

Nutrition:

Carbohydrates – 4.6 g

Fiber – 1.2 g

Fat – 0.4 g

Protein – 1.5 g

Calories – 25

260. Hawaiian Salsa

Preparation Time: 20 minutes

Cooking Time: 0 minutes

Servings: 6

Ingredients:

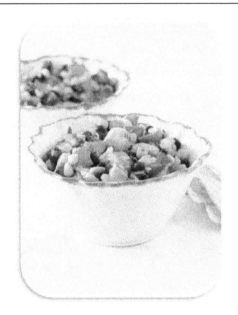

- 4 fully ripened tomatoes, diced
- ½ sweet onion, diced
- ½ cup fresh mango, diced
- ½ cup pineapple, diced
- ¼ cup apple cider vinegar
- ½ tsp sea salt

Directions:

1. In a large airtight container, mix together all ingredients.

2. Cover and chill for 15 minutes so the flavors blend before serving.

Nutrition:

Carbohydrates – 5.3 g

Fiber – 1.4 g

Fat – 0.2 g

Protein – 0.9 g

Calories – 48

261. Great Gravy

Preparation Time: 5 minutes

Cooking Time: 10 minutes

Servings: 6

Ingredients:

- 1 Tbsp coconut oil, melted
- 2 Tbsp coconut flour
- ½ cup vegetable broth
- 2 Tbsp almond milk
- ½ tsp sea salt

Directions:

1. In a saucepan over medium heat, heat the coconut oil. Don't let it get too hot or the flour will instantly burn.
2. Add the coconut flour and whisk to make a thick paste.
3. Slowly whisk in the vegetable broth. Bring to a boil and cook for 4 minutes, or until thickened.
4. Reduce the heat to low. Add the almond milk and salt. Continue cooking until the desired consistency.
5. Serve warm.

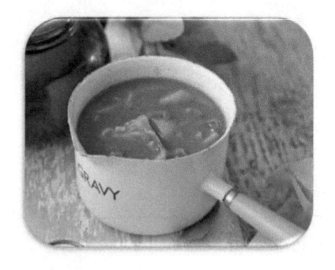

Nutrition:

Carbohydrates – 2.8 g

Fiber – 0.8 g

Fat – 2.5 g

Protein – 1.8 g

Calories – 35

262. Apple Butter

Nutrition:

Carbohydrates – 12.9 g

Fiber – 1.9 g

Fat – 0.2 g

Protein – 0.2 g

Calories – 49

Preparation Time: 10 minutes

Cooking Time: 3 hours

Servings: 24

Ingredients:

- 4 pounds apples, peeled, chopped
- 2 cups fresh apple juice
- 1 Tbsp lemon juice, freshly squeezed
- 2 packets stevia
- 1 tsp cinnamon
- 1 vanilla bean, split lengthwise, deseeded
- Pinch ground cloves

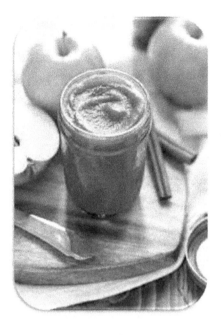

Directions:

1. Add the apples, apple juice, and lemon juice to a pot. Bring to a simmer and cook for 1 hour, until soft. Remove from the heat and cool slightly.
2. In a blender, purée the apples until smooth.
3. Take the puree out. Add the stevia, cinnamon, vanilla bean seeds, and cloves to the apples. Cook for an additional 2 hours, stirring frequently.
4. Cool the apple butter. Transfer to an airtight container and refrigerate.

Nutrition:

Carbohydrates 12.9 g – Fiber 1.9 g – Fat 0.2 g - Protein 0.2 g - Calories 49

263. Sun-Dried Tomato Sauce

Preparation Time: 10 minutes

Cooking Time: 0 minutes

Servings: 4

Ingredients:

- 1 cup cherry tomatoes, halved
- ½ cup tightly packed sun-dried tomatoes
- 3 Tbsp coconut oil
- 1/3 cup fresh basil
- 1 Tbsp tomato paste
- 1 tsp sea salt
- 1 tsp garlic powder

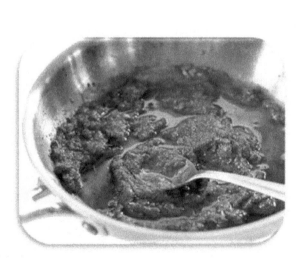

Directions:

1. In a food processor, combine all ingredients.
2. Pulse to combine. Serve.

264. Enchilada Sauce

Preparation Time: 5 minutes

Cooking Time: 26 minutes

Servings: 8

Ingredients:

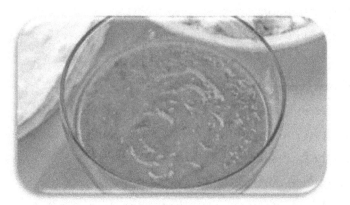

- 2 Tbsp coconut oil
- 2 Tbsp coconut flour
- 2 Tbsp chili powder
- 2 cups water
- 1 8-oz can tomato paste
- 1 tsp garlic powder
- ½ tsp cumin
- ½ tsp onion powder
- ½ tsp sea salt
- ¼ tsp red pepper flakes

Directions:

1. In a pot over medium heat, heat the coconut oil, coconut flour, and chili powder. Cook for 1 minute.
2. Add the water, tomato paste, garlic powder, cumin, onion powder, salt, and red pepper flakes, to taste. Bring the mixture to a simmer and cook for 25 minutes, stirring occasionally.
3. Serve warm.

Nutrition:

Carbohydrates – 8.3 g

Fiber – 1.6 g

Fat – 3.6 g

Protein – 1.8 g

Calories – 68

30 Day Meal Plan

Day	Breakfast	Lunch	Dinner	Snacks/Desserts
1	Good Morning Popeye	Chicken-Sausage Frittata With Corn And Feta Recipe	Carrot and Golden Beet Soup	Baked Apples
2	Garden Pancakes	Alkaline Cauliflower Fried Rice	Sweet Potato Green Soup	Berries Granita
3	Tropical Granola	Creamy Avocado Cilantro Lime Dressing Recipe	Lentil Spinach Soup	Pumpkin Ice Cream
4	Summer Fruit Salad with Lime & Mint	Creamy Avocado Dressing	Tangy Lentil Soup	Lemon Sorbet
5	Winter Fruit Compote with Figs & Ginger	Southwestern Avocado Salad Dressing	Vegetable Casserole	Avocado Pudding
6	All-American Apple Pie	Brain Boosting Smoothie Recipe	Mushroom Leek Soup	Chocolate Mousse
7	Baby Potato Home Fries	Lemon Avocado Salad Dressing	Red Lentil Squash Soup	Blueberry Crumble
8	Breakfast Fajitas	Avocado Salad With Bell Pepper And Tomatoes	Cauliflower Potato Curry	Apple Crisp
9	Brown Rice Porridge	Avocado Egg Salad	Vegetable Bean Curry	Coconut Macaroons
10	Spaghetti Squash Hash Browns	Avocado Caprese Salad	Wild mushroom soup	Chickpea Fudge

11	Salad in Your Hand	Avocado Salmon Salad With Arugula	Quinoa, Bean, & Mango Salad	Pumpkin spice crackers
12	Warm Spinach Salad	Alkaline Spaghetti Squash Recipe	Mixed Bean Salad	Spicy roasted nuts
13	Salad on a Stick	Tomato & Greens Salad	Quinoa & Lentil Soup	Wheat Crackers
14	Emeraland Forest Salad	Cucumber & Onion Salad	Lentil & Veggie Soup	Potato Chips
15	Summer Dinner Salad	Apple Salad	Mixed Mushroom Stew	Zucchini Pepper Chips
16	Roasted Vegetable Salad	Cauliflower Soup	Veggie Stew	Apple Chips
17	Quinoa & Avocado Salad	Tomato Soup	Bean & Veggie Chili	Carrot Chips
18	Avocado-Caprese Salad	Asparagus Soup	Lentil Chili	Pita Chips
19	Spicy Sesame Noodle Salad	Okra Curry	Kidney Bean Curry	Sweet Potato Chips
20	Organic Baby Tomato & Kale Salad	Eggplant Curry	Pumpkin Curry	Pumpkin spice crackers
21	The Asian Bowl	Garlicky Broccoli	Tofu with Broccoli	Chocolate Milkshake
22	The Breakup Bowl	Sautéed Kale	Black-Eyed Pea Curry	Strawberry Gazpacho

23	The Fight It Off Bowl	Parsley Mushrooms	Chickpea Mashed Potatoes	Tomato Salsa
24	The Hawaiian Bowl	Vegetarian Burgers	Mushroom And Onion Gravy	Avocado Guacamole
25	The Indian Bowl	Carrot and Golden Beet Soup	Vegetable Chili	Cauliflower Hummus
26	The Italian Bowl	Sweet Potato Green Soup	Spinach With Chickpeas And Lemon	Kale Chips
27	The Mexican Bowl	Lentil Spinach Soup	Raw Green Veggie Soup	Quinoa Porridge
28	The Rose Bowl	Tangy Lentil Soup	Kale Caesar Salad	Apple Quinoa
29	The Southern Bowl	Vegetable Casserole	Red And White Salad	Kamut Porridge
30	Simple Bread	Mushroom Leek Soup	Almond Milk	Hot Kamut With Peaches, Walnuts, And Coconut

This is an example of a 30-day Meal Plan, according to the alkaline diet. You can choose your favorite recipes from this cookbook and modify some of these with what you like best.

Conclusion

One of the biggest problems we're facing today is the low quality of food, as processed foods bombard us, and natural food is not accessible to everyone. Whether we're talking about restaurants or supermarkets, processed food is abundant. Around 70% of the diseases known today are caused by the food we eat, and we have to thank processed food for this. This type of food is very low in nutritional value and has all sorts of chemicals and added sugars harmful to your body. This is how we end up with high blood pressure, heart disease, type 2 diabetes, kidney stones, liver disease, or even more severe cancer. When it comes to processed food, everything is about profits, which means high quantity and low quality. Especially because of the mass-production techniques spawned by the Industrial Revolution philosophies, the poor quality of grains, fruits, and vegetables are accumulated in animals that eat those same poor agricultural products. Thus, the human diet consists of compounding layers of poor food quality. **The alkaline diet emphasizes balancing the pH level in your body**. This indicator is the measurement unit for the ratio between the acid and alkaline levels in your body. Processed food has a very high acid level, and this leads to serious diseases. The alkaline diet aims to lower the acid level and increase the alkaline level to prevent such diseases and conditions. *The alkaline diet encourages you to eat mostly veggies and fruits, which by default are more alkaline than acid.*

The 30-day plan included in this book can lead you in the right direction. It encourages the consumption of fruits, veggies, and seeds, which are known to flush out toxins, lower blood pressure, and lower the risks of type 2 diabetes, heart disease, and cancer. Vegetables, fruits, and seeds can easily provide the nutrients your body requires, so you will not lack anything, and you will not be hungry. The alkaline diet is not designed as a weight loss program, but instead, it focuses on improving your overall health. To make sure the alkaline diet is working, you will need to purchase the right food, follow sound alkaline-based recipes, cook healthy food, and chew the food properly to make it easier for the digestive system to do its job. Also, you may need to work out, as any diet combined with physical exercise can maximize the results related to health and weight loss. This 30-day Alkaline Meal Plan doesn't need any special medical approval, as it's not a drastic diet which can cause harmful effects for people with different health conditions, but it can be tried by anyone who wishes to eat healthy, to feel more energized and to avoid different medical conditions and diseases. It is designed to cover your daily macronutrient needs, so your body can function properly. Get started today with the 30-day meal plan for a fresh and solid start on the path to improving your health! Even though the plan is for just 30 days, you will definitely feel the difference and you can stick to this plan for as long as possible.

I hope the recipes you found in this book could help your health and your body! Thanks for reading!

CPSIA information can be obtained
at www.ICGtesting.com
Printed in the USA
BVHW051121301220
596746BV00009B/496